THE POWER OF

female health, fertility & pregnancy

THE KNOWLEDGE

THE POWER OF
female health, fertility & pregnancy

BY DR NIGHAT ARIF

hamlyn

hamlyn

First published as *The Power of Female Health, Fertility & Pregnancy*
in Great Britain in 2025 by Hamlyn, an imprint of
Octopus Publishing Group Ltd
Carmelite House
50 Victoria Embankment
London EC4Y 0DZ
www.octopusbooks.co.uk

An Hachette UK Company
www.hachette.co.uk

The authorized representative in the EEA is Hachette Ireland,
8 Castlecourt Centre, Dublin 15, D15 XTP3, Ireland (email: info@hbgi.ie)

This material was previously published as *The Knowledge:
Your guide to female health from menstruation to the menopause* by Aster in 2023

Text copyright © Dr Nighat Arif 2025

With thanks to The Cleveland Clinic Foundation for reference images used
on pages 167 and 169.

ISBN 978-0-60063-972-5
eISBN 978-0-60063-973-2

A CIP catalogue record for this book is available from the British Library.

Typeset in 10.5/15pt Sabon LT Pro by Six Red Marbles UK, Thetford, Norfolk

Printed and bound in Great Britain.

1 3 5 7 9 10 8 6 4 2

This FSC® label means that materials used for the product have
been responsibly sourced.

MIX
Paper | Supporting
responsible forestry
FSC® C104740

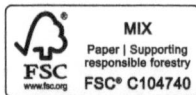

Disclaimer: Before making any changes in your health regime, or starting any
medical treatment, always consult your own doctor for advice relevant to
your individual circumstances.

Staff Credits:
Publisher: Kate Fox
Senior Editor: Pauline Bache
Art Director: Jaz Bahra
Words Contributor: Joanne Lake
Illustrator: Liliana Rasmussen
Picture Research: Giulia Hetherington and Jennifer Veall
Copy Editor: Joanne Smith
Production Manager: Caroline Alberti

CONTENTS

YOUR GUIDE TO FEMALE HEALTH

Back in the spring of 2019, I was working at a practice in rural Buckinghamshire as a GP with a special interest in women's health. That area of medicine had always fascinated me, from menstruation through to menopause, and helping people to access the right care and treatment had become my vocation and my passion.

Alongside my GP duties, I began to create social media posts to raise awareness of various topics: the importance of cervical screening, for instance, or the benefits of HRT. I wanted to use my experience as a clinician to empower women with knowledge, to encourage them to get to know their bodies and to dispel the myths that were often perpetuated within the area of women's health. To communicate these important messages in the most effective manner possible, I took great care to use clear language, factual terminology and evidence-based data. Furthermore, as someone with Pakistani heritage, I was keen to reach out to a South Asian audience, so I produced content in Urdu and Punjabi as well as English.

My tweets, TikTok and Instagram posts began to gather momentum and soon caught the attention of the BBC. In May 2019, they invited me onto the show to discuss the common symptoms of menopause and my efforts to raise awareness in the ethnic minority community. This appearance by a 30-something, hijab-wearing Muslim woman caused quite a stir, not just because I was talking openly about night sweats and vaginal dryness – considered taboo subjects by many – on a flagship TV programme, but also because GPs who looked like me were rarely seen on TV. The positive feedback I received as a consequence – especially from women of colour – completely blew me away.

More TV appearances followed (including on ITV) and my social media hits skyrocketed. I received thousands of responses from people across the globe who had watched one of my videos, recognized their own symptoms and – armed with new-found information – had checked in with a healthcare professional. As a GP this was music to my ears, of course, but it also highlighted a huge demand for clear, factual and accessible advice. And that, in a nutshell, is what prompted me to grab my laptop and write *The Knowledge*.

I want to share my expertise. I want to start a conversation. I want you to understand your body, to identify any changes and to realize when – and how – to seek help. Ultimately, I want you to look after yourself in the best way possible so you can lead a long, happy and healthy life. It is so important to me that women of all ages are able to advocate for themselves and get the best healthcare possible. So this series of books will cover women through every stage of life, from Puberty, to their Fertile Years, into Midlife and beyond. However, there are some elements of female health that truly do transcend the ages – I'm thinking of the need to understand your body, know your rights, and be aware of lifelong health checks.

So, this essential information is included at the front of all books in this series – to provide a comprehensive guide to female health at every stage of life.

I firmly believe that everyone assigned female at birth, regardless of age, should learn about the three distinct phases and the changes they embrace. Indeed, during the writing process I found it helpful to view things from the perspective of my 14-year-old self. I was raised in a traditional, religious Muslim household where women's health matters were hardly discussed, so I had to use other means to learn about things like menstruation and contraception. The teenage 'me' would have undoubtedly appreciated a book like this, as it would have given me a deeper understanding of myself . . . and a deeper understanding of my mother and grandmother!

And while I want to help women and girls of all ages, I'm just as keen to help their loved ones, too – that's mums, dads, siblings, grandparents and other relatives or caregivers. I particularly want to reach out to fathers, perhaps those who are single, separated or widowed – or in same-sex relationships – who may not have female partners to consult. It's so important that you feel comfortable talking to your daughters about period products, or family planning, and can do so openly and honestly.

Removing the shame and stigma from women's health is an ongoing mission of mine and forms a central theme of these books. The embarrassment factor can prove to be fatal, quite literally, if it prevents someone from getting the right care at the right time. Gynaecological cancers claim thousands of lives each year but, by performing self examinations of your breast tissue, vulva and vagina – and having regular smear tests – any changes or anomalies may be spotted early enough for you to obtain successful treatment. We also need to encourage our children and young people to familiarize themselves with their genitals without feeling ashamed. By normalizing these matters – girls checking their vulvas, boys checking their penises – good habits will be formed and infection and disease may be averted. So much of my work as a GP involves this kind of preventative care; it genuinely does save lives.

This series also offers help and advice for individuals who don't fit the mould of what society – and the healthcare system – still deem as 'normal' (although I always question this concept, because in medicine there's no such thing as a 'normal' period, for example, or a 'normal' menopause). I'm very proud of the fact that this book includes guidance for trans people and those with disabilities. These individuals have exactly the same rights to sexual and reproductive healthcare as any other patient, and should receive treatment without discrimination or prejudice. This content may also be useful to fellow clinicians, who should be ensuring their surgeries and consultations are as inclusive and as accessible as possible.

I apply a similar principle to people struggling with infertility or baby loss, whose circumstances should never be overlooked or underplayed. Successful conception, pregnancy and childbirth is still very much part of the common narrative, meaning that those who encounter

4

problems often feel excluded from the conversation. Many women of colour can feel side-lined, too; institutional racism, combined with systemic misogyny, continues to prevail in the healthcare sector and I still hear appalling stories from women of colour whose symptoms are dismissed and whose pain is invalidated. I'm determined to combat this, and will continue to call for allies to fight our corner and for ambassadors to connect with communities.

And let me be clear: should anyone query why inclusivity, diversity and ally-ship is so important to me, and why it forms such an intrinsic part of my ethos (and this book), I'll always flip it around to ask, 'Well, why shouldn't it be important? And why should the question even need to be asked in the first place?' As far as I'm concerned, the basic principles of medicine are universal. Gold-standard healthcare should be available to all. No one should face bias or exclusion; on the contrary, they should all have a place at the table.

As a member of an ethnic group, and an employee of the UK's National Health Service (NHS), the issue of representation really matters to me. It's a known fact that most promotional healthcare material – leaflets, posters, diagrams and illustrations – does not always feature people of colour. This, quite understandably, can send the wrong signals to people who may already feel excluded from mainstream medicine, and who are therefore less likely to engage with clinicians. I'm doing my utmost to challenge and change this, and am immensely proud of the illustrations that have been specially created for this book. I only wish they'd existed when I was younger; back then, public health messaging was distinctly white, Western and middle class.

I'm also keen to break down the cultural barriers that prevent women of colour from accessing the care they need. Many of their health issues, including menstruation and menopause, are kept 'under the veil' (not spoken about, in other words), which can have a severe impact on their wellbeing. To these people – and to anybody else who's feeling alone and isolated – I truly hope I can help you to find your voice and start that conversation.

But along with being heard, you also need to feel seen. And as someone who eats, sleeps and breathes clinical medicine, I want all women to know that I see them, whether suffering with endometriosis, living with perimenopause, coping with infertility, struggling with gender identity, or simply wanting to be sure that their periods are normal. This book, I hope, will empower you to get the healthcare you deserve and, not only that, will encourage you to spread the word and tell your story. Your knowledge is a gift, to be shared freely with others. I hope this book plays a role in providing a pillar of support on that journey. You may not find every single answer within these pages – medicine is rarely one-size-fits-all, and no two people experience the same symptoms – but if you spot a nugget of advice that prompts you to pick up the phone to your doctor, or encourages you to perform your first self examination, then this labour of love will have served its purpose.

Finally, each one of us carries a candle of knowledge. Kindled by wisdom and experience, it brings light, warmth and energy. But we shouldn't keep the candle to ourselves. We should use it to light somebody else's. That way, the flame continues to burn brightly.

With love,

Nighat Arif

Dr Nighat Arif

Dear body, thank you for harbouring me, making me beautiful, nourishing me, making me capable of remarkable things. I promise to love and respect you.

FEMALE ANATOMY & SELF EXAMINATIONS

Awareness of your own body is key to good health, so it's vital that you educate yourself about your basic anatomy, both internal and external. In every book in this series, I have included the following pages with diagrams of the internal female reproductive system and breasts, as well as a diagram of the external vulva and pubic area. These should really help as a reference point for many sections of the book that follow.

While much of your internal anatomy won't be visible to you, it is still vital that you have a keen awareness of how areas of your body look and feel – because every body is different, only you can know your own body best. If I had my own way, every woman or person assigned female at birth (AFAB) would examine their breast tissue and genitals on a regular basis from the age of 13. Ideally, by the time you are 18, you should complete all self examinations once a month, in between periods. The more we learn about the way we look, and the way things feel, the more likely we'll be to notice changes and spot anomalies. Flagging up any concerns to your doctor may help them recognize certain symptoms and make early (sometimes life-saving) diagnoses. Pages 19–23 and 31–5 will show you how to undertake these self examinations in detail.

The female reproductive system

The female reproductive system includes everything involved in creating and carrying a baby, but it is so important to have an awareness of your system at every stage of your life, even if you never intend to have a pregnancy. The system begins at the vulva, the external element that you can see in your self examination (see pages 14–15), then moves into the vagina and then the cervix, which is the opening to the uterus. The uterus is lined with the endometrium and is where, if you are pregnant, the foetus will grow and be supported throughout your pregnancy. If you are not pregnant, then your menstrual cycle runs through a process of thickening the endometrium and then shedding the lining with your period. The ovaries are where an egg (ovum) matures each month, which is then released into the fallopian tube to travel along towards the uterus.

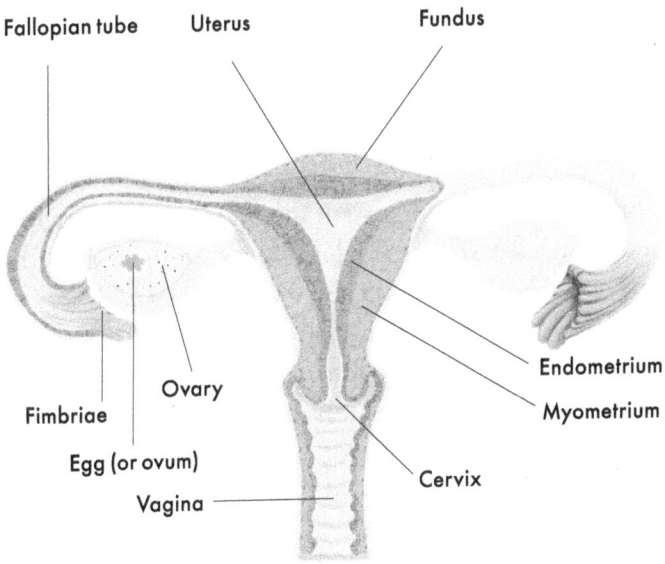

Fallopian tube

Uterus

Fundus

Fimbriae

Ovary

Egg (or ovum)

Vagina

Cervix

Endometrium

Myometrium

The female reproductive system (side view)

People are frequently surprised by how close the reproductive system is to the lower part of the digestive system, but they are all snugly clustered together within the pelvis. This is particularly important to note during times when your natural levels of the hormone oestrogen drop, as this is the reason why vaginal atrophy (see *The Power of Menopause & Midlife*) can cause infections in the urinary tract. Your bladder and urethra sit just in front of your uterus and labia, while the bowel, rectum and anus sit just behind. Between the lower opening of the vulva and the anus is an area called the perineum, which can easily split or become sore if the skin becomes dry.

FEMALE ANATOMY & SELF EXAMINATIONS

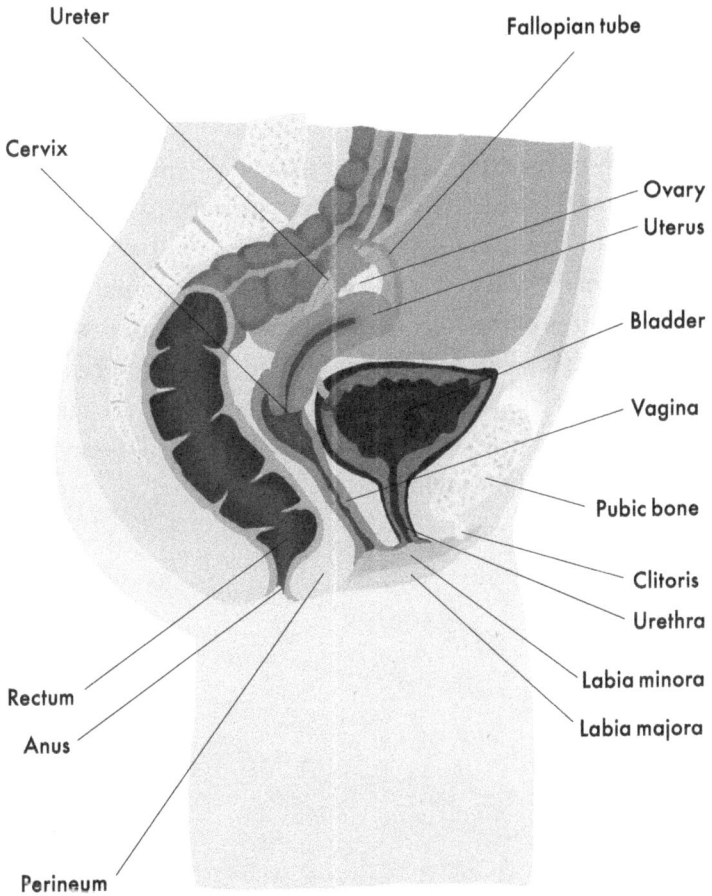

Ureter

Fallopian tube

Cervix

Ovary

Uterus

Bladder

Vagina

Pubic bone

Clitoris

Urethra

Labia minora

Labia majora

Rectum

Anus

Perineum

The vulva & pubic area

The vulva is the external part of your genitals while the pubic area is that between your legs, above your vulva, where your pubic hair grows. Looking into the vulva you will see that it's formed of the outer labia and inner labia. The clitoral hood sits at the top of the inner labia and covers the clitoris, while the urethral opening (where you urinate from) is just below. The entrance to the vagina sits at the bottom of the inner labia, then the perineum is the area of skin that sits between the openings of the vagina and the anus.

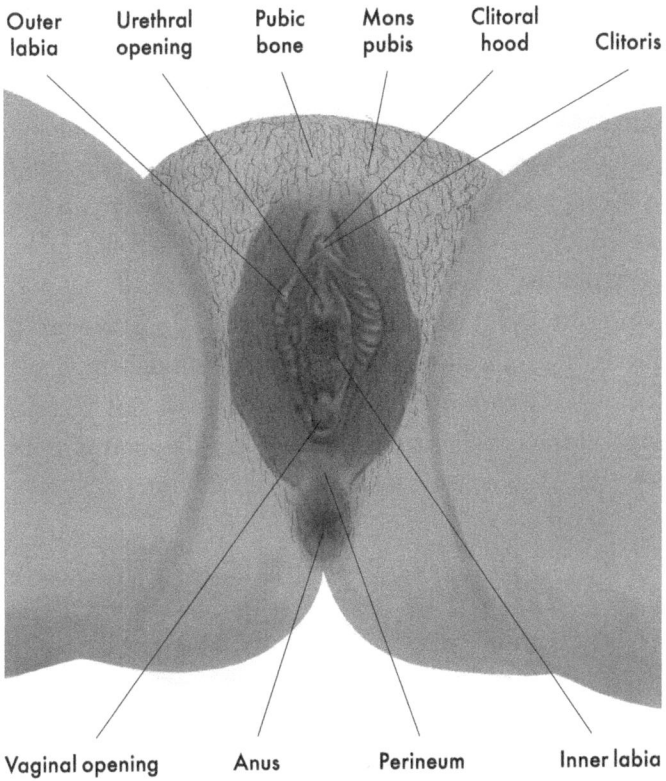

Outer labia

Urethral opening

Pubic bone

Mons pubis

Clitoral hood

Clitoris

Vaginal opening

Anus

Perineum

Inner labia

The breast

The breasts sit in front of the chest, separated from your ribs by the pectoral muscles. Each breast is formed of several lobules (or alveoli), around 15 to 20 in each breast, that are connected via milk ducts and milk reservoirs to tiny openings in the nipple. The hormonal changes associated with late pregnancy and childbirth will stimulate the alveoli to make milk and the action of a baby suckling at the breast will cause a 'let down', when the milk is released from the alveoli, through the milk ducts and reservoirs out through the nipple openings. The first milk that comes from the breast is a rich, fatty substance called colostrum and then the 'mature' milk is produced about two days after a baby is born.

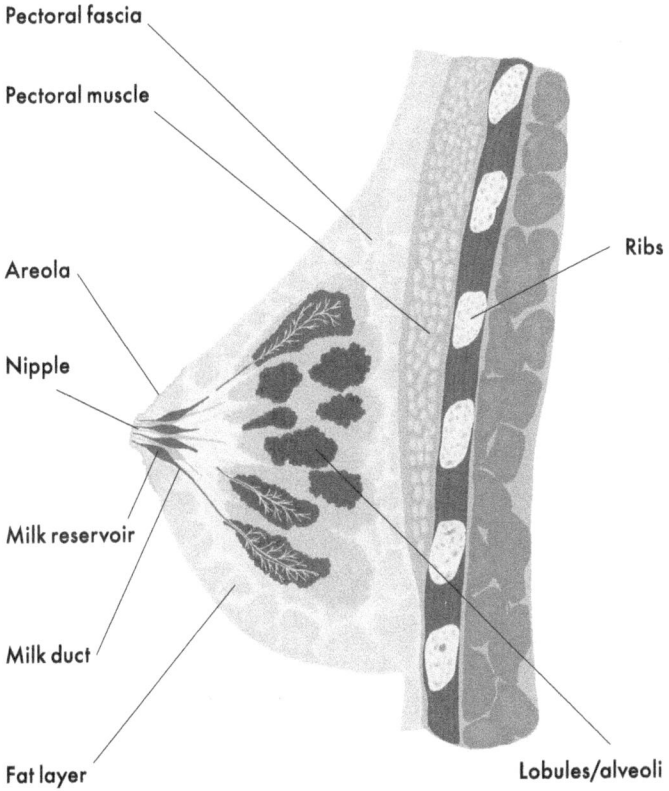

Pectoral fascia

Pectoral muscle

Areola

Nipple

Milk reservoir

Milk duct

Fat layer

Ribs

Lobules/alveoli

SELF EXAMINATION: BREASTS

Breast cancer is very common and, in the UK, about one in seven women will be diagnosed with it in their lifetime. Early detection significantly improves the chance of successful treatment and recovery, which is why it is so important to examine your breast tissue on a regular basis. Thanks to the increased raising of awareness throughout the NHS – and the fabulous work of charities like Breast Cancer Now – more women are examining their breast tissue than ever before. A thorough self examination should take about ten minutes and might just save your life.

Examining your breasts

I advise my patients to do breast examinations on a monthly basis: on roughly the same date each month, or two weeks before or after your period if you're menstruating (as fluctuations in oestrogen around your period are likely to cause breast pain and swelling that might mean missing any lumps).

Perform your breast exam wherever it feels comfortable (preferably somewhere nice and quiet, where you won't be disturbed) – perhaps on your bed, or in the bath or shower. I often tell my patients to do it at a particular time of day, which might help to jog their memory and make it a routine, perhaps in front of their bedroom mirror as they're getting dressed for work on a Monday morning. I know some women who ask their partners to have a good feel of their breast tissue – you'd be surprised how many lumps are found by loved ones – and you can always return the favour by assisting with their personal examinations. It's important to point out that those assigned male at birth can get breast cancer too, so it's a good idea for them to check their pecs regularly.

Breast implants can make a self examination more difficult but it is still important. You should be able to gently shift the position of the implant and you can then palpate around the implant to feel the breast tissue around it.

What to look out for during a breast self examination

- A new lump in the breast or armpit area, which may or may not cause pain.
- Irritation, redness, darkening or flaking of the skin around the breast and nipple area.
- A swelling or thickening in any part of the breast.
- Skin snagging, puckering or dimpling around the nipple area.
- Nipple discharge or blood if not pregnant or nursing.
- A marked and visible change in breast size (it's common for women to have one breast bigger than the other, but watch out for *recent* changes).
- A dull or sharp pain in any area of the breast.

Try to focus and concentrate as you feel your breasts. Don't be half-hearted or absent-minded! Remind yourself that you're feeling for lumps and bumps in the breast tissue and armpit area, and are looking for any changes in the skin or nipple.

If you *do* notice any irregularities during a self examination, try not to panic or assume the worst. Make a note of these changes, however small, and book an appointment to see your doctor as soon as possible, outlining the reasons to the receptionist when you call.

Do not delay matters or tell yourself that you're worrying unnecessarily. The sooner you get seen by a clinician, the better. And – should anything require further investigation – you'll be promptly referred to a specialist.

How to examine your breasts

Examine your breast tissue monthly, preferably between your periods. Find somewhere you are comfortable, either standing up or lying on your back. Then remove your top and bra. Complete the following steps on both sides.

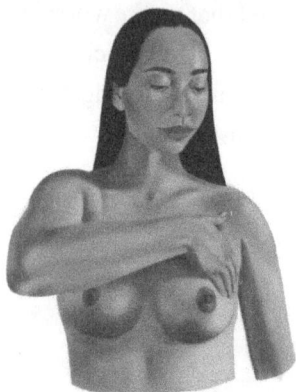

1 With the pads of four fingers, slowly press around the fleshy breast tissue in a circular motion, moving outwards from the nipple to your rib and armpit areas. Apply pressure that's firm, but comfortable. Feel for any changes to the flesh or skin as outlined opposite.

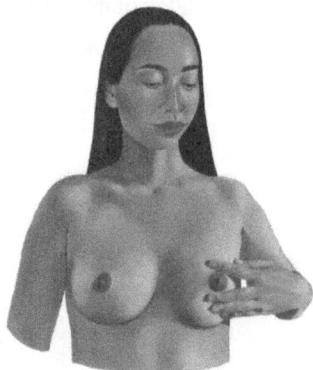

2 Use your fingers to feel underneath and around the nipple, looking for any changes to the flesh or skin.

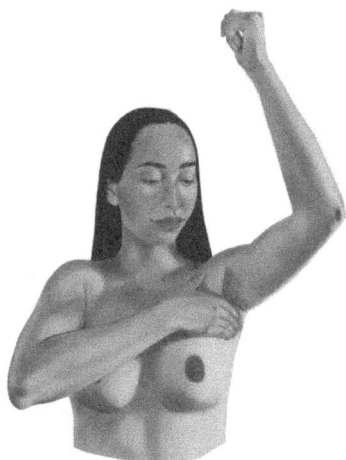

3 Use your fingers to feel underneath the armpit, looking for any changes to the flesh or skin.

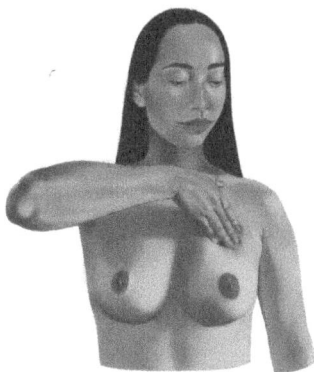

4 Walk your fingers up your chest towards your neck, feeling as you go, looking for any changes to the flesh or skin.

WEAR THE CORRECT SIZE BRA!

see so many women in my surgery with chronic breast pain who are clearly wearing the wrong-sized bra. When I was younger, I never received any guidance about the importance of wearing the right bra. I was none the wiser until the age of 23, when a lovely lady in the lingerie department of a local shop introduced me to the joys (and comfort) of wearing a correctly fitted bra!

The easiest way to find your bra size is to visit the lingerie section of your local department store, or a stand-alone lingerie store. The staff there will be specially trained in measuring busts. Many bra-fitters now determine your size on sight, without a tape measure – a real specialist skill! If, however, you don't feel comfortable visiting a store, or can't find the time to, then you can measure yourself at home, and calculate your bra size from there.

How to measure your bra size

You'll need to take two measurements to determine your bra size: the band measurement and the cup measurement. If possible measure in inches (because that's how bra sizes are calculated), but you can use an online calculator to convert from centimetres if your tape measure doesn't show inches.

To find the band size, measure all around your ribcage just beneath your breasts. (If the measurement is an odd number then scale up or down to the nearest even number.)

This number is your band size. Then measure all around the widest area of your bust, so the tape measure sits firmly but comfortably. Subtracting your band size from this bust measurement will give your cup size, so less than 1 inch (2.5cm) = AA, 1 inch (2.5cm) = A, 2 inches (5cm) = B, 3 inches (7.5cm) = C, 4 inches (10cm) = D, 5 inches (12.7cm) = DD, 6 inches (15.2cm) = E, 7 inches (17.8cm) = F, 8 inches (20.3cm) = FF, 9 inches (22.9cm) = G, 10 inches (25.4cm) = GG, 11 inches (27.9cm) = H. Sizes beyond H are usually available from specialist retailers.

What to look for in a well-fitting bra

- It should be snug when on the loosest hook.
- The shoulder strap should sit comfortably to prevent shoulder pain.
- The cups should be flush with your bust.
- The centre wire or fabric should sit flat against the chest wall; if it pulls away the cup is not deep enough, and if it wobbles the cup is too deep.
- At the sides, the bra wire or fabric should sit under the breast along the ribs; if it sits on the breast tissue, the cup is too small, and if the side wire is too big it will dig into the underarm area.

Cup size = measurement 1 minus measurement 2

How to measure your bra size

Find somewhere you can measure yourself comfortably without being distracted, then either measure over a soft (non-padded) bra – whichever bra you currently find most comfortable to wear – or against your bare breasts.

1 Measure the circumference around the fullest part of your breasts (shown by the solid line in the image on page 29). The tape measure should have a little give in this measurement.

2 Measure the circumference around your ribcage beneath your breasts (shown by the dotted line in the image on page 29). The tape measure should be very snug, but still comfortable for this measurement.

3 Calculate your bra size using the formula on page 26.

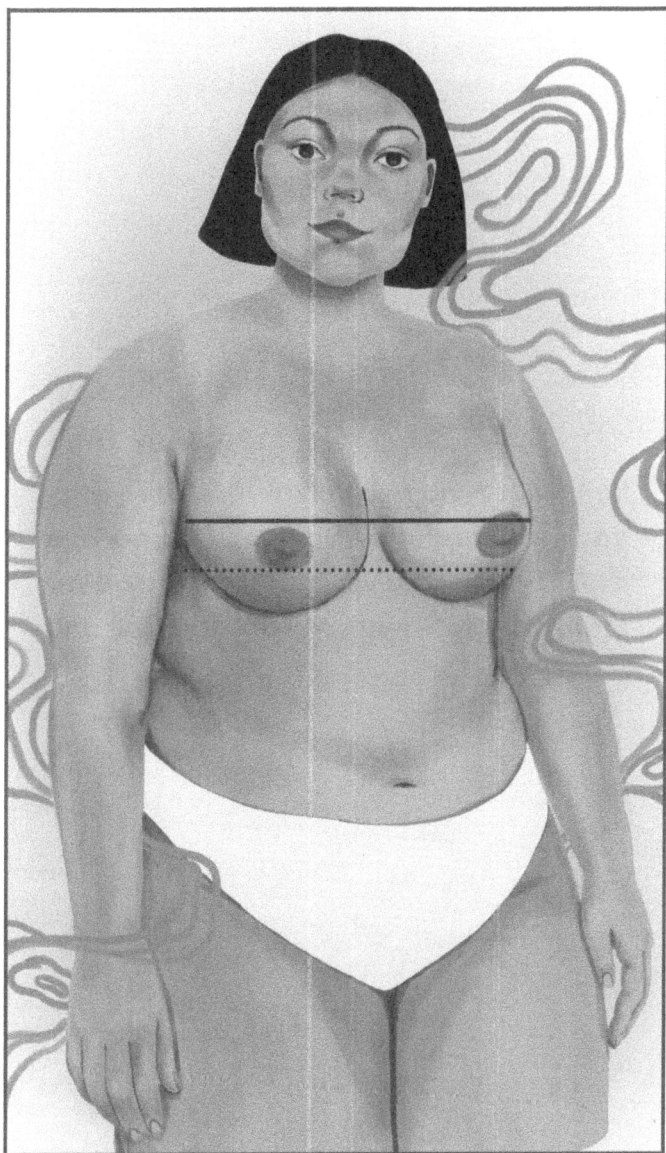

Remember: no two vulvas look the same, each is completely unique. And no one should know your vulva and vagina better than you. So why not grab a mirror and get started?

SELF EXAMINATION: VULVA & PUBIC AREA

Whilst breast self examinations have become commonplace – and have saved countless lives – there is still a huge lack of awareness around genital self examinations. This simply has to change if we are going to reduce the incidence of vaginal and vulval cancers, so it is vital you familiarize yourself with your vulva and pubic area.

Examining your vulva & pubic area

Vulval and vaginal cancers are rare but frequently missed or misdiagnosed (see page 173). They can occur in women of any age, more often among those who are long-term smokers or who have a family history of melanoma (a type of skin cancer). There are 1,400 new cases of vulval cancer each year in the UK and five every week of vaginal cancer. While they are awful diseases, if picked up early, then the prognoses are encouraging. Self examination is key and, as per usual, this is a euphemism-free zone, so no talk of foo-foos or front bottoms whatsoever!

Not to be confused with the vagina, the vulva is another name for your external genitals, namely the labia majora (outer lips), the labia minora (inner lips) and the clitoris. Speaking as a doctor who has examined thousands of women, I can assure you that no two vulvas look alike.

Becoming familiar with the way your vulva looks and feels is very, very important.

If we're going to raise awareness about vulval examinations, however, we first have to remove the stigma and take away the sexualization of women's bodies in today's society. Examining and touching your vulva for health purposes isn't remotely pornographic – it's a sensible thing to do, not a sexual thing to do – and we need the men in our lives to respect and support us in this regard.

We also need to reach the stage where we can encourage our children to regularly examine their genitals without embarrassment. By normalizing things – girls checking their vulvas every week, boys checking their penises and testicles – good habits will be formed and infections and diseases may be recognized and treated at an early stage.

A vulval examination should ideally take place monthly: on roughly the same date each month, similarly to a breast examination (I often encourage my patients to get into the routine of doing the examinations one after the other). You'll need some privacy – and won't want interruptions, of course – so perhaps choose a locked bathroom or bedroom, preferably with some natural light. Find yourself a small hand-held mirror, and set aside ten minutes or so.

What to look out for during a vulva & pubic region self examination

- Any lumps, bumps, spots or sores that could indicate infection, disease or other conditions.

- Any changes to the colour or size of different areas from one examination to the next.
- Any bad-smelling discharge (though some discharge is normal, and the amount will depend on what point you are at in your menstrual cycle). If your discharge has a bad smell or is an unusual colour (see *The Power of Puberty & Periods*) it could indicate an infection.

How to examine your vulva & pubic region

Examine your vulva monthly, preferably between your menstrual periods, if you have them. Before you begin, wash your hands with soap and water, then grab a hand-held mirror and find somewhere with enough space to sit, squat or lie down, on the floor or on a chair, and sufficient light for you to see well, where you won't be interrupted for ten minutes.

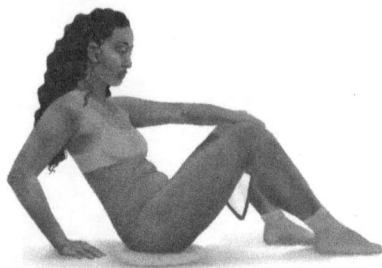

1 Open your legs and check the area where your pubic hair grows. Feel around with your fingers and position your mirror to check for moles, bumps, spots, warts, ulcers, lesions, rashes or white patches. Make a mental note of anything that looks new or feels different. Examine the fleshy area from top to bottom.

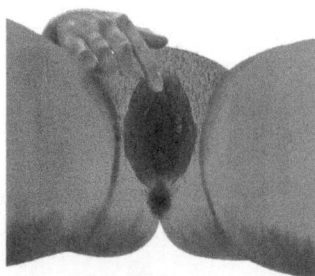

2 Next, find your clitoris – at the top of the vulva, the fold of skin where the inner labia meet – and look for any bumps, growths or discolouration.

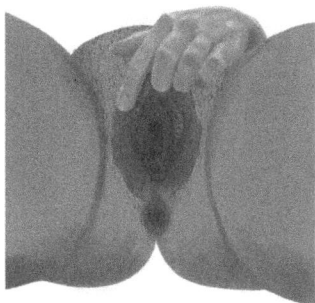

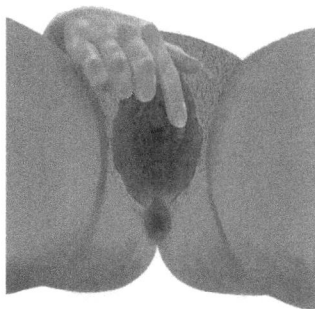

3 Check your labia majora – the outer lips – and, again, feel for any bumps, spots, lesions or rashes.

4 Check your labia minora – the inner lips – and, again, feel for any bumps, spots, lesions or rashes.

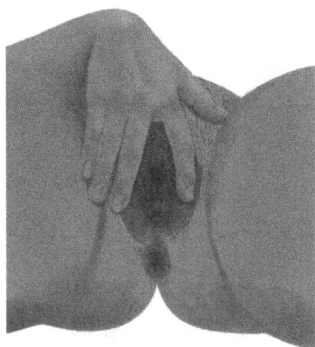

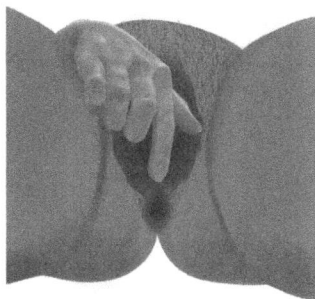

5 Prop the mirror in front of you and use one hand to gently hold open your labia minora, to see into your vagina. Check your vagina for any bumps, spots, lesions or rashes. You may see what look like 'rings' going around the vaginal wall – this is called mucosal tissue and is completely normal.

6 Finally, check your perineum (the area located between the entrance to the vagina and the anus) for any lumps, bumps or anomalies. When you have finished, wash your hands again. Make a note of any changes detected and, if you're at all worried about any anomalies, don't hesitate to consult your doctor for a professional examination.

FAIR HEALTHCARE ACCESS FOR ALL

I feel strongly that everybody – whatever their creed, colour, background, ability or gender expression – should have equal access to healthcare when they visit my surgery or any other service in the healthcare system.

However, this is still not the case for many people trying to access healthcare and advice. Patients can be discriminated against for many reasons and access to fair healthcare for ethnic minorities, those who are disabled and the LGBTQ+ community is woefully below the ideal standard. In order to counterbalance this, and to ensure that such disparity and discrimination is eradicated, we need allies to help fight our corner, and ambassadors to try to connect with our communities.

ETHNIC MINORITIES

Institutional racism and systemic misogyny continue to prevail in healthcare, to the detriment of ethnic minority women. The health issues of women of colour are often dismissed by clinicians or their own community, and their pain is downplayed and invalidated.

In some ethnic minority communities, when someone is unwell they're more likely to have a mindset of 'I will be cured if I pray hard enough' or 'this is a test of my faith'. This can lead to a reticence to address any symptoms with a doctor, and the shame and stigma persists. Women are also less likely to discuss women's health matters with others in their community – whether that's talking about examining themselves, or about a lump they've found – and this inhibits vital information sharing. It's really important for us to recognize this issue within ethnic minority communities, and to realize that more health advocates are needed in situ to raise awareness and strengthen messages.

I'm all too aware that, among Black and Asian ethnic minorities, there's still a lot of shame and stigma around breast examinations, for example. Within some parts of society – particularly faith-based communities – breasts are highly sexualized, prompting the mindset that they're something to keep hidden. This often deters women from checking their breasts at home, or having them examined by a doctor. Whatever their symptoms, ethnic minority women are also more likely to wait for an appointment with a female doctor which, due to sheer demand, can lead to a delay. If you have an immediate health concern you may be seen much quicker by a male doctor, who will be more than happy to offer you a chaperone, or let a friend or family member accompany you.

When you make a medical appointment, don't be afraid to state your preferences:

- If you feel uncomfortable being seen by a doctor of a particular gender, you may state your preference to the receptionist.
- Ask to bring someone with you to your appointment (a friend or family member) or, alternatively, you can put in an advance request for the surgery to provide a chaperone; this might be another health professional.

All doctor's surgeries will offer you a chaperone during an appointment if you prefer, or will let you take a friend or family member with you.

If English isn't your first language, and none of the doctors happen to speak your first language, you can ask the receptionist to book an interpreter for you or, if you prefer, take someone to the appointment who can translate for you.

Removing barriers

Language can be a significant obstacle for women whose mother tongue is Urdu or Punjabi, for example, and who are unable to see a doctor who speaks it. Talking about menopause or other women's health issues can be embarrassing enough for these patients, but saying 'my night sweats soak my sheets' or 'sex with my husband is really painful' via a family chaperone or an interpreter can be problematic. In order to address these issues, not only do we need a more ethnically diverse workforce in the healthcare sector, we also need Western-trained doctors (myself included) to recognize these cultural barriers.

A lack of understanding about women's health can prevent ethnic minority women from accessing the care they need. It's become a personal mission of mine to target more evidence-based information at these hard-to-reach communities, and I regularly post short videos and longer-form interviews and Q&As on social media. Most of my posts on TikTok, Twitter and Instagram are spoken or subtitled in Urdu and Punjabi, as I've realized that many women in those communities will respond much better to verbal rather than written information (illiteracy levels are particularly high among first-generation South Asian female migrants). My social media feeds share the same handle – @DrNighatArif – so please feel free to watch and share.

If English isn't your first language, you can ask for a translator if necessary (although you may have to be quite insistent).

Improving representation

Most healthcare-related promotional material – including many leaflets, posters and illustrations – does not feature people of colour. This can send the wrong message to ethnic minorities who feel excluded from mainstream medicine and are less likely to engage with healthcare professionals.

I'm doing my utmost to try to change this. In 2019 I worked with the Pausitivity campaign group to produce a #KnowYourMenopause poster in Urdu, specifically aimed at connecting with midlife women in South Asian communities. Being the first of its kind, the poster had a massive impact when it was distributed to doctors' surgeries and community centres across the UK. A poster was also produced in Welsh, too.

Over the last few years I've also had the privilege of appearing on TV including the BBC and ITV to discuss medical matters, often from a women's health perspective, which range from hot flushes to vaginal dryness. The response from my South Asian sisters has been overwhelmingly positive. They appreciate watching someone on TV who speaks for them and looks like them; let's be honest, there aren't many Muslim women wearing pink hijabs on national TV! There's no doubt about it . . . representation matters.

8.9% of residents of England and Wales did not have English as their main language in 2021

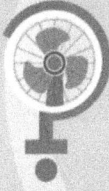
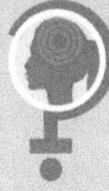
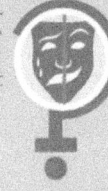
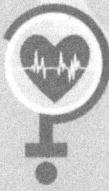
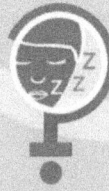
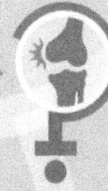
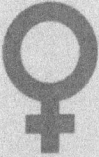

My 2019 collaboration with Pausitivity, which produced posters in Urdu to raise awareness of menopause symptoms in the South Asian community. The Pausitivity team also produced a Welsh-language poster to increase awareness in Welsh-speaking communities. Posters reproduced with thanks to Elizabeth Carr-Ellis and the Pausitivity team.

WOMEN'S HEALTH & DISABILITY

n order to reduce barriers to healthcare, doctors should make their surgeries and consultations as accessible as possible, and we should be acting as ambassadors and allies for all patients.

A 2021 article entitled 'Barriers in access to healthcare for women with disabilities' in the *BMC Women's Health* journal stated that 'women with disabilities (WWD) are more likely to have unmet healthcare needs than women without disabilities'. This statement was corroborated by the following findings outlined by the Sisters of Frida organization, a collective of disabled women:

- Disabled women have limited access to prenatal care and reproductive health services.
- Most maternity care does not meet the needs of disabled women.
- Disabled, older, asylum-seeking and Traveller women face obstacles in accessing healthcare.

In my own practice, I strive to ensure that all of my patients with physical disabilities receive the same healthcare as my able-bodied patients, and I will consider certain practicalities, such as adapting the way I fit a wheelchair user with a coil, or discussing which period products might suit their circumstances. I'll always outline the risks and benefits to an individual so they are in total control of their decision; empowering my patients is what I'm here for! If a patient is visually impaired, I'll often record voice notes, instead of writing things down or printing things out.

I also tend to use audio-based instructions for anyone who has difficulties with reading; summarizing their contraceptive options via voice notes on their phone, for instance, will always optimize healthcare for these people more than a factsheet or website. Patients with hearing loss are welcome to attend my consultations with a British Sign Language (BSL) interpreter. This is often a friend or family member but outside of this, the options are sadly limited. (A free remote interpreting service – BSL Health Access – was set up in 2020 to enable deaf people to access phone consultations but, at the time of writing, is sadly no longer funded.) Clarity of communication is vitally important when you're discussing life-changing decisions, and I hope this barrier will be removed soon.

Consultations can also be complex if I'm seeing a patient with a cognitive impairment, perhaps associated with a condition like Down's syndrome or Huntington's disease, or with neurodiverse conditions. In these instances, the way in which I communicate their healthcare options, and the way I obtain medical consent, often has to be adjusted. While I'll endeavour to involve the patient as much as possible, if they are unable to make cognitive decisions about fertility or contraception, for example, I may choose to consult with the person who has the patient's best interests at heart and who can make a decision on their behalf, often a parent, sibling or guardian.

These are just some ideas for how the healthcare system can work for all, and I hope these ideas will empower you to request the adjustments *you* may need to get the best healthcare for you, and your family too.

Become your own advocate. Get informed, do your research, become empowered and DO NOT accept discriminatory behaviour.

RIGHTS FOR TRANS PATIENTS
(& ADVICE FOR THEIR DOCTORS)

F ear and apprehension can often deter trans people from seeing their doctor. This is a heart-breaking situation that can have potentially harmful consequences.

The 2018 Stonewall *LGBT in Britain Health Report* stated that, while there are 'committed individuals and organizations doing outstanding work' in the NHS and beyond, it is also true that 'instances of discrimination, hostility and unfair treatment in healthcare services are still commonplace'. Indeed, three in five trans people (62 per cent) said they'd experienced a lack of understanding of specific trans health needs by healthcare staff.

In 2021, the TransActual organization conducted their Trans Lives survey, a cross-sectional study that recorded the experiences of trans people, including those of colour and those with disabilities. Their findings were truly depressing. Fourteen per cent of respondents had been refused medical care on at least one occasion, on account of being trans. Fifty-seven per cent of trans people – that's more than half – said they had avoided going to the doctor when unwell. Fifty-three per cent of trans people of colour experienced racism while accessing trans-specific healthcare services, and 60 per cent of disabled respondents reported suffering ableism in similar circumstances.

So how can the GP experience be improved for trans

patients? Luckily, significant steps are possible to overcome those barriers and optimize their healthcare and the majority of healthcare professionals are inclusive and supportive of such adaptations and changes. The following advice, I hope, will be helpful to both patients *and* clinicians.

Changing your name & gender details

Any patient can change their name and gender on their doctor's medical records, and this can be done as an informal decision for those under the age of 16 (before they can legally change their name via deed poll). An individual can also state their preferred pronouns, whether it's he/him, she/her or they/them, for example. Surgeries should have a specific form for this purpose, which can usually be provided by the admin team. Your details will be updated on the practice IT network, and will appear on your doctor's computer screen, so there should be no need to 'explain' yourself at an appointment, which can be upsetting. More recently I've got into the habit of asking all my patients to confirm their preferred pronouns; I think it's quite an empowering thing to do.

Surgery trans policy

Ideally, your surgery will have a trans health policy and, even better, a practitioner who has a specialist interest in trans healthcare who will be best placed to understand your emotional and physical needs. For those doctors who feel their knowledge is lacking in this area – or needs updating – there are many opportunities for further learning and continual professional development and I'd like to encourage all doctors (and people!) to be aware of trans issues and how they can affect the individuals concerned.

Routine cancer screening

When a trans person changes their gender details, they are often issued with a new NHS number. It's really important to obtain confirmation from the doctor's surgery that your data has been migrated successfully so that you'll continue to receive invites for national cancer screening programmes.

Trans men, trans women and non-binary people aged 50-plus should receive an invite for a mammogram if they have breast tissue (due to either naturally occurring oestrogen or oestrogen hormone replacement). A trans man with a uterus will need to attend a cervical smear test every three years between the ages of 25 and 49, and every five years after that until they are 65.

Trans people who've changed their gender marker may not necessarily receive automatic call and recall invites for the relevant cancer screenings so please check that you've not been missed off any lists by flagging this with your healthcare provider. Ideally, there should be a member of staff with sole responsibility for keeping track of the trans patients in the recall system; my own practice has a nurse dedicated to that very task.

It's vital that trans people don't miss out on cancer screening. Double-check with your doctor that you're in the system.

Gender identity clinic referral

I hear many cases of trans people being met with ignorance, even hostility, when they've requested a referral to a gender identity, or gender dysphoria clinic (GDC), perhaps to access gender-specific counselling, medical or surgical affirming therapy, or hormone therapy. This situation requires specialist care, and patients should expect to be treated with dignity and respect before being signposted accordingly (see *The Power of Puberty & Periods* for referral options). There is also plenty of valuable guidance for doctors on the General Medical Council website, including shared care agreements and bridging prescriptions.

Shared care agreements

Some adult trans people (those over the age of 18) choose to access private healthcare for their hormone therapy – often because the waiting list for NHS clinics is so long (often years rather than months). I advise anyone doing this to diligently keep notes of your treatment as, by pursuing the private route, you are in effect becoming your own care-giver (you'll have to monitor your own blood hormone levels, for example).

You can, however, ask your GP to draw up a 'shared-care agreement' that allows an exchange of information between your private clinic and your doctor's surgery. Having these notes to hand will enable your GP to help with any issues associated with your hormone therapy, such as disrupted menstruation, clitoral growth, increased libido, increased facial and body hair (for trans men); or reduced facial and body hair, lower libido, decreased sexual function and genital shrinkage (for trans women).

Bridging prescriptions

In certain circumstances, adult trans patients who are waiting for treatment at a gender identity clinic can benefit from 'bridging' prescriptions. General Medical Council guidance currently allows GPs (preferably in collaboration with the gender identity clinic) to prescribe hormone treatment to patients who are suffering physically and/or psychologically as they wait for an appointment. In normal circumstances – outside of the bridging prescription remit – GPs are not usually expected to prescribe hormones to trans people unless they have the expertise and knowledge required.

As this has no impact on NHS budgets – hormones are relatively cheap, after all – many clinicians see this as discriminatory. My fellow GP, Dr Kamilla Kamaruddin, is a passionate advocate for trans health and is among those who find this situation problematic. When we last caught up she questioned the fact that GPs could give hormone treatment to cisgender males who had hypogonadism (a condition that can cause erectile dysfunction), the safety profile for which is similar to prescribing testosterone treatment to trans-masculine people, and GPs could also prescribe gonadotropin-releasing hormones to cisgender male patients with prostate cancer, and to cisgender females with endometriosis, but some GPs were reluctant to prescribe hormones to trans patients under a shared-care prescribing agreement with the GDC.

Complaints procedure

Each surgery has a complaints procedure. If you experience any form of intolerance or discrimination from a doctor, or a member of surgery staff, or if your GP has done nothing to help you, you should report it. You can either register a complaint with your practice manager or contact your local health authority (this advice applies to patients across the board, of course). You are also entitled to request to see a different doctor within your practice, and you can switch your surgery without having to provide a reason. Your local LGBTQ+ group may be able to suggest a more suitable alternative.

When people gain useful knowledge and information about their health issues, they'll go around sprinkling it like confetti . . .

FEMALE HEALTH, FERTILITY & PREGNANCY

INTRODUCTION

Planning for a baby can be one of the most thrilling times of your life. Introducing a little person into your household, along with all the love and happiness it will (hopefully) bring, can be a joyful prospect. So, if you've decided to take the plunge . . . many congratulations, and may I wish you all the luck in the world!

Starting a family is such a momentous decision and, of course, there are lots of things to consider beforehand. 'Only have a baby when you're ready' is the advice I often give to my patients. Have a long, hard think about whether it's a sensible decision for all involved, and ask yourself a few important questions:

- Is it the right time for you to get pregnant?
- Are you in good health?
- Will you be able to juggle your home life with your work life?
- Can you afford childcare?
- Do you have a decent support network?
- Is your relationship in a good place?

Indeed, if you do have a partner, please ensure that you're both ready and willing to go down this route. I've faced awkward situations in my surgery when one half of the couple isn't sold on the idea of having a baby, unbeknownst to the other. I remember one patient whispering to me that they were secretly using contraception as they weren't ready for the patter of tiny feet!

As for timing your pregnancy, it's commonly known that your best reproductive years from a biological standpoint are in your twenties, when your ovaries store the highest number of good-quality eggs, and when your pregnancy risks are at their lowest. Fertility begins to decline gradually during your thirties – particularly after the age of 35 – but that doesn't mean you can't become pregnant during that time or beyond. Depending on lifestyle and other factors, there's no reason why women in their thirties, maybe up to their mid-forties, can't go on to give birth to healthy babies.

However, as someone who's dealt with all manner of fertility and pregnancy-related issues – and as a mother of three myself – I've learned you have to start managing your expectations. Despite your best efforts and intentions, you cannot schedule in a baby. Like buses, they'll come when they want to (and sometimes it can be two or three at once!). The journey towards pregnancy can be erratic and unpredictable and you may have to prepare yourself for lots of twists, turns and bumps in the road. Things may not always go quite to plan, and the whole process can often be fraught with stress, worry and confusion.

Prospective parents who come to my surgery always have lots of questions – rightly so; it's a life-changing decision – and I hope this part of the book provides you with a few answers, as well as some useful tips and advice.

In this chapter I'll be looking at fertility and pregnancy issues through a family doctor's lens, which means I'll be outlining the most common cases and conditions we face in general practice. More specific issues that might ordinarily be addressed by your midwife, gynaecologist or obstetrician, therefore, may not be covered in depth. With this in mind, check out the Resources section to help you find excellent sources of information about the second and third pregnancy trimesters, as well as the birth itself.

This section of the book will largely refer to male and female partnerships, but I'm mindful that families come in all configurations. Indeed, some of the happiest, healthiest and well-cared-for children who visit my surgery belong to single-parent families, or belong to parents from the LGBTQ+ community. These people should receive the same level of care and support as anybody else, of course, so much of my advice will apply to them. The NHS offers information for transgender and non-binary pregnant people and other health authorities should too (see Resources from page 203).

Towards the end of this section I'll also be covering other health considerations that people of child-bearing age need to be aware of, such as health screening and recognizing symptoms of gynaecological cancer.

PLANNING FOR PREGNANCY

I f you've set your heart on becoming pregnant, my advice is to plan ahead, gather as much information as you can and get yourself in the best possible shape. If you're in a relationship, the latter applies to your partner, too – the fitter and healthier you both are, the more likely you'll conceive. Ideally, you should try to make the following changes to your health and lifestyle.

Dietary supplements & lifestyle changes

It is important to ensure your baby gets adequate nutrients from the point of conception. A healthy, varied diet should be complemented by nutritional supplements and a healthy lifestyle.

Take folic acid

Folic acid reduces the baby's chances of having neural tube defects (NTDs) such as spina bifida. One to three months before you begin trying to conceive you should take 400 micrograms (0.4 milligrams) of folic acid every day, and for at least 12 weeks after conception. Current recommendations actually advise women to continue taking it throughout pregnancy and during breastfeeding, too. You may take 5,000 micrograms (5.0 milligrams) of folic acid if you or the other biological parent has a neural tube defect, if you've previously had a pregnancy affected by an NTD, have diabetes, or you or your partner takes anti-epilepsy medication.

Take vitamins

All pregnant individuals should take 10 micrograms (400iu) of vitamin D throughout their pregnancy and while breastfeeding. However, be careful to avoid multivitamins that contain vitamin A (retinol), as too much of this in the first trimester can harm the baby's development by affecting the nervous and cardiovascular systems and, in rare cases, trigger spontaneous miscarriage. It is also advisable to avoid liver and liver products (including fish liver oil) during this time as they contain high levels of vitamin A.

Stop smoking

Smoking cigarettes during pregnancy is linked to miscarriage, high levels of premature birth, low birth weight and sudden infant death syndrome (SIDS). The baby also has an increased chance of having breathing problems in the first six months of life. Quitting the habit can be hard, I know, but it's the sensible thing to do for you and your baby. Luckily, there is so much support out there, including the free NHS Quit Smoking app that you can download onto your phone (see Resources from page 203). The app allows you to track your progress, offers you motivational support, and even shows you how much money you're saving. According to NHS data, if you can make it to 28 days without smoking, you're five times more likely to quit for good!

Stop drinking

Alcohol guidance for pregnant women has changed a great deal over the years. Gone are the days when you were encouraged to drink a famous Irish stout! As it stands, current guidance recommends that alcohol should be completely avoided, since it increases the risk of miscarriage, premature birth and low birth weight. Drinking heavily during pregnancy may also cause your baby to develop foetal alcohol spectrum disorder (FASD), a serious condition that can lead to lifelong issues.

Judging by those who visit my surgery, the vast majority choose to stick to a no-alcohol rule while they're pregnant. I know some women find it hard to kick the 'wine o'clock' habit, but there are many great alcohol-free drinks available to try. My personal favourites include alcohol-free gin with tonic and zero-alcohol beer (fab with a curry!).

Review your medications

Always check with your doctor that any medication you have been prescribed is safe to take during pregnancy. There has been some controversy surrounding sodium valproate, a drug that treats conditions such as epilepsy and bipolar disorder, since it's said to have caused birth defects and developmental problems. As far as I'm concerned, this medication should *never* be prescribed to women of child-bearing age but, in the event that it is, it should only be given to those taking contraceptives. Don't hesitate to raise any concerns about sodium valproate with your doctor.

Avoid recreational drugs

You must stop using recreational drugs such as cocaine and cannabis, both before and after your pregnancy. Substance and/or alcohol abuse can affect a parent's ability to look after their child, and can cause real danger if they fall asleep next to an infant (there have been tragic cases of babies being accidentally suffocated when a drowsy parent rolls over in the middle of the night).

Stick to a healthy weight

It's always very sensible to keep to a healthy weight, whatever stage of life you're at, but this is particularly important if you're trying to conceive.

If you're overweight with a BMI (body mass index) above 30, you may have issues conceiving or responding to fertility treatment. You also have an increased risk of miscarriage (see page 93), high blood pressure, deep vein thrombosis (DVT) and gestational diabetes (see page 105). Before you become pregnant, I advise you to use a BMI calculator to keep track of your weight and also to consider using a health and fitness app or website. There are some brilliant options out there, many available for free (see Resources from page 203).

> To calculate your body mass index, divide your weight in kilograms by your height in metres squared (or use an online calculator!)
> $BMI = kg/m^2$.

If you're underweight with a BMI below 18.5, you may be more likely to experience hormonal imbalances that could affect ovulation and may affect your chances of getting pregnant. I have many underweight patients who go on to have healthy babies, but having a low BMI can put you at a higher risk of miscarriage, and can increase your chances of having a premature birth (when the baby is born before it is fully developed), an underweight baby, or a baby that suffers with gastroschisis (a condition whereby the baby's stomach does not develop properly).

If you have an underlying eating disorder that may be contributing to your low weight, please talk to your doctor about arranging a prenatal assessment. There is also a great deal of practical support available from charities and other organizations (see Resources from page 203).

Check your vaccinations

It's vital to ensure that you're up to date with your vaccinations. Having your MMR (measles, mumps and rubella) jab is particularly important, because rubella – commonly known as German measles – can harm your baby if you contract it while pregnant, particularly in the early stages. If you're unsure about your immunization history, speak to your health practitioner who will be able to access your medical records or carry out a blood test to check your rubella immunity. And, if you're given the MMR jab, you should avoid becoming pregnant within one month of the vaccine.

One of the most common questions I'm asked by pregnant people is, 'Should I have the Covid-19 vaccination?' My answer is a categorical *yes*. In April 2021, the RCOG (Royal College of Obstetricians and Gynaecologists) and the JCVI (Joint Committee on Vaccination and Immunization) concluded that the Covid-19 jab was safe and could be given at any time during pregnancy, but preferably after the first trimester. I firmly believe that if you're offered the vaccine, you should take it, as pregnant women who contract Covid-19 are more likely to have complications from it (although they are at no greater risk of being infected in the first place). Data shows that one in five pregnant women who have become unwell with the virus give birth early so, by having the vaccine, mums-to-be will be safeguarding themselves from going into premature labour. Not only that, the vaccine also provides immunity to the baby against Covid-19.

Underlying conditions
If you have one of the following long-term underlying conditions, you'll be put under the care of a specialist consultant obstetrician for the duration of your pregnancy, alongside your midwife care, as your pregnancy will be considered higher risk:

- Diabetes
- High blood pressure
- A heart condition (or previous heart condition)
- Thyroid issues

- Cancer
- Mental health conditions

Routinely, anyone with Afro-Caribbean, Mediterranean, Indian, Pakistani, Southeast Asian and Middle Eastern heritage should be offered a screening test for two inherited blood disorders – sickle cell disease and thalassemia. You can also ask for a free test from your doctor if you're worried you might be predisposed to these conditions.

Sexually transmitted diseases
Depending on your sexual history – whether you've had unprotected sex, for example – you and your partner may want to book yourselves in for an STD review before you begin trying for a baby. You can make an appointment at your local sexual health clinic where you'll be tested and treated for free, with the utmost confidentiality.

When left untreated, some STDs can affect you and the developing baby – a gonorrhoea infection (see *The Power of Puberty & Periods*), for example, can lead to miscarriage, premature birth, low birth weight and chorioamnionitis (a bacterial infection of the membranes that surround the foetus and the amniotic fluid in which the baby floats). Gonorrhoea can also affect the baby as it passes through the birth canal and, if left untreated, can cause eye infections in the child.

STDs can also cause scarring and blockage of the male and female reproductive structures. If they remain untreated in women, this can lead to an episode of pelvic inflammatory disease (PID, see page 159), which is a leading cause of infertility.

Increasing your chances of conceiving

Conception is such an inexact science. It's impossible to say how long it will take a woman to become pregnant, because so much depends on the circumstances of each individual and each couple. The fortunate among us will become pregnant straight away, while others will take longer or, very sadly, will never be able to conceive by 'natural' methods. According to NHS figures, 92 per cent of women aged between 19 and 26 will conceive within one year, and 98 per cent will conceive within two years. If you're aged between 35 and 39, 82 per cent will conceive within one year and 90 per cent within two years.

However, in order to maximize your chances of conceiving, I'd suggest, in the first instance, you should follow the tips on planning for pregnancy I've outlined above. Once all that's in place, it's time for the fun bit! Having regular sexual intercourse is an essential part of conception, of course, particularly around the time that the woman is ovulating (releasing an egg). There are a number of ways you can monitor this:

- **Track your cycle** using an app or a diary (ovulation occurs about 14 days after your period starts).
- **Record your body temperature** with a thermometer (it rises up to a degree during ovulation).

- **Use an ovulation test kit** (this detects any increase in the luteinizing hormone in your urine).
- **Keep an eye on your normal vaginal mucus** (it might be wetter, clearer or more 'slippery' at the time of ovulation).
- **Take note of any breast tenderness,** breast swelling, abdominal pain or bloating (these can also be signs of ovulation, but working it out this way is not always that accurate).

The National Institute for Health and Care Excellence (NICE) guidance suggests you should have good-quality vaginal sex (with ejaculation) with your partner every two or three days, without contraception. Contrary to popular belief, daily intercourse isn't always a good idea because it can lead to a decrease in sperm concentration. And, forgive me for stating the obvious, but always ensure the sperm enters the vagina!

Fertility problems

Statistically, one in seven couples will experience fertility related problems that create an obstacle to achieving parenthood. If you've not conceived successfully after one year of unprotected sex, on average, there may be an underlying problem that needs further investigation. Having problems conceiving is a very normal occurrence, but this doesn't make it any less distressing. You may think you've ticked all the boxes – having regular sex, following a healthy lifestyle – yet that dreaded period keeps arriving every month, like an unwelcome visitor. In these circumstances, there's no harm in visiting your doctor to talk things through and assess your situation. If you're in a relationship, I think it's really important to address these issues together. Emotions can run high on both sides – there's often a lot of guilt, anxiety and frustration – but, in order to reach your goal, you and your partner will need to support one another. It takes two to make a baby, after all.

1 in 7 couples in the UK are affected by infertility

Society still places blame at the woman's feet, but it's understood that 50 per cent of cases are specifically related to male fertility problems (usually the result of a low sperm count). Other fertility problems could be associated with at least one of these factors:

- Age
- Sexual intercourse quality or frequency; regular sex means unprotected vaginal sex at least every two to three days.
- Physical disorders: obesity, anorexia, breathing problems, cardiovascular issues.
- Sexually transmitted diseases (STDs).
- Hormonal problems such as polycystic ovary syndrome (PCOS), early menopause and issues with thyroid or pituitary glands.

- Reproductive system problems, such as pelvic inflammatory disease (PID), blocked fallopian tubes, adenomyosis and endometriosis.

It's the latter two issues – hormonal and reproductive system complications – that I'd like to focus on here. I see many patients in my surgery whose fertility is affected by these problems, and I'm keen to do all I can to raise awareness.

INFERTILITY (& YOUR OPTIONS)

Around one in seven couples are unable to conceive naturally. Sometimes this is due to known hormonal or reproductive issues but sometimes – despite a succession of tests, scans and examinations – the problem remains unexplained.

If you and your partner are healthy, having unprotected sex and have been unable to conceive a child after trying for one year, you should both see your doctor. They will discuss possible ways forward with you, and will outline a number of options. The good news is that many infertile people *can* go on to become parents. Thanks to the wonders of modern medicine and specialist intervention, up to 80 per cent of couples (or single parents) are able to have children.

Getting the basics right

Healthy lifestyle habits will help create optimum conditions, and it's important to remember that these should apply to *both* potential parents, as sperm quality and quantity can be harmed by an unhealthy lifestyle.

- **Try to keep to a healthy weight** – have plenty of exercise and ensure you have a good diet. Sometimes it's helpful to have a prenatal discussion with your doctor to look at weight reduction (or weight gain).
- **Cut out smoking** as there are absolutely no benefits!

- **Cut down alcohol** consumption as much as possible.
- **Have regular unprotected sex** at least twice a week.
- **Manage your anxiety and stress;** trying to get pregnant can be an anxious time as a couple, so you might consider cognitive behavioural therapy (CBT).
- **Keep track of your ovulation window** using a luteinizing hormone kit.

Getting help if you're having difficulty becoming pregnant

Firstly, book an appointment with your family doctor. Most appointments are only ten minutes long, so try to book a double (20-minute) appointment for you and your partner. During this appointment, your doctor will discuss your situation and medical history. This may include questions about your lifestyle, but may also include some very intimate questions about your sexual and gynaecological history.

The doctor might also perform a physical examination, perhaps a bi-manual exam for the female (sometimes using a plastic speculum) and a testicular examination for the male. Your doctor may also order the following tests:

- Baseline health check for both partners.
- Full blood count.
- Kidney, thyroid and liver function.
- Cholesterol check and diabetes check.
- Chlamydia test.
- Progesterone/gonadotropins check (female partner).

- A referral for a transvaginal ultrasound scan of the uterus, ovaries and fallopian tubes (female partner).
- A sperm analysis (male partner).

Medical procedures to improve female fertility

Following your doctor's initial investigations, you will be referred directly to a hospital's obstetrics and gynaecology department in order to establish the underlying reason for infertility. From then on, family doctors will not prescribe or instigate any fertility medications themselves, but we will often have conversations with patients about the various options they might be offered by their hospital consultant.

Medical options to improve female fertility include the following medications:

- **Metformin**, which is used in women with PCOS to help with insulin resistance and assist weight loss.
- **Clomifene citrate (clomid)**, which can help to regulate ovulation in women who have irregular periods.
- **Gonadotropins**, which can help to stimulate ovulation, and also help with male infertility.

These medications can have side effects, and giving ovulation-stimulating drugs to couples with unexplained infertility is not recommended unless under specialist guidance.

Surgical procedures to improve female fertility

Once you've been assessed, if the issues affecting your fertility have been identified, you may be referred for surgical procedures to correct the issue. Surgical procedures to improve female fertility include the following:

- **Fallopian tube surgery** can be performed to correct any blockages or scarring found in the fallopian tubes. The success of the surgery depends on the extent of the blockage or scarring in the tubes.
- **Laparoscopic surgery** investigates whether endometriosis or PCOS is affecting your chances of getting pregnant. If there is endometriosis, and adhesions are noticed, then adhesiolysis (cutting away of the lesions) can help with pain and can assist with pregnancy (see page 150).
- **Ovarian drilling** is a laparoscopic surgical procedure that involves drilling away the ovarian cysts that have formed as a result of PCOS; this can help when ovulation-stimulating medication has not.

Assisted conception

Assisted conception refers to a range of specialist treatments, including intra-uterine insemination (IUI) and in-vitro fertilization (IVF), that can help a patient to get pregnant. If my patients are interested in obtaining fertility treatments on the NHS, I'll suggest they read the relevant NICE guidelines as the availability of IUI and IVF is dependent on the funding of your local Integrated Care Boards (ICBs). These tend to follow the criteria below and are usually only available to couples who do not already have children:

- Three IVF cycles for women who are under the age of 40, and who've been trying for two years.
- One IVF cycle for women who are aged between 40 and 42.

The main assisted conception options for those in heterosexual relationships who are struggling to become pregnant, same-sex couples or those who wish to start a single-parent family, are listed below:

- **Intra-uterine insemination (IUI)** is the procedure whereby sperm is directly placed into the uterus (this could be your partner's sperm or donated sperm). This may take place if vaginal intercourse is not possible, or may be an option for same-sex couples. Ordinarily, same-sex couples can have six cycles of IUI and, if they don't become pregnant, will need to look at private options. Indeed, some couples pay for their treatment anyway because NHS waiting times for IUI are extremely long.
- **In-vitro fertilization (IVF)** is a process in which the egg is fertilized with sperm in a laboratory and then placed into the uterus. The egg and sperm can belong to the couple, or can be donated. The process of IVF is extremely intense and may not always be successful – younger women are more likely to have a successful assisted pregnancy, and IVF is not recommended by the NHS for women older than 42 (for that reason, many decide to seek private treatment). I always

advise my patients to try to remain positive, but also to prepare themselves for a lot of stress and anxiety (and financial hardship). Getting the right advice and support is crucial, as is doing your research. See Resources from page 203 for more information.

There are six stages of IVF:

1 Suppression of natural menstrual cycle, involving daily medication to stop the normal cycle and expel the uterus lining.

2 Stimulation of ovulation, involving daily medication to encourage extra eggs to be released by the ovaries. During stimulation, ultrasound scans are performed every 1–3 days to check the progress of the maturation of the eggs.

3 Preparation for egg collection, involving a single dose of human chorionic gonatrophin (hCG) medication given at a precise time once scans show the eggs are ready for collection. You will be given an exact time for your egg collection in the next 24 hours.

4 Egg collection, a procedure during which a long, thin needle is put into the vagina and the eggs are harvested from the lining of the uterus.

5 Fertilization, a process when the retrieved eggs are mixed with the sperm in a laboratory test tube for a few days to allow fertilization.

6 Transfer of embryo: the fertilized embryos are placed back in the uterus. Usually you will be asked to wait two weeks before taking a pregnancy test.

Other considerations

There are a number of other areas of fertility treatment and help that can be used alongside I V F and I U I. These include:

- **Egg/sperm donation**, which involves someone donating their eggs or sperm to people who are unable to use their own to become pregnant. If you have female- or male-factor infertility you may find donated eggs or sperm will help you. I would always advise patients to use a licensed clinic where the sperm and eggs are carefully screened for sexually transmitted diseases and/or genetic disorders. Reputable clinics will also provide appropriate legal advice to their clients. Alternatively, you may wish to donate yourself. Helping others in this way is such a wonderful, selfless thing to do, and there are now many NHS schemes that allow people to donate.
- **Egg preservation/egg harvesting/egg freezing** is a method that takes unfertilized eggs from the ovaries and freezes them, preserving them for future use.

Alternative routes to parenthood

Medical and surgical procedures aren't suitable, or successful, for everyone. Many people become parents by surrogacy or adoption, while others may choose to become foster carers. Living child-free – out of choice or circumstance – is a perfectly reasonable alternative, too.

Your body has not failed you because you didn't fall pregnant 'naturally'.

LGBTQ+ PARENTS & ASSISTED CONCEPTION

More and more members of the LGBTQ+ community are choosing to become parents these days. Society has changed, thank goodness – hooray for diversity and equality! – and families now come in all shapes and sizes. Anyone who wants to have children should of course receive the same care and consideration from healthcare professionals, regardless of their sexual preference or gender identity.

Many lesbian couples (or single people) I see in my surgery choose to conceive via sperm donor insemination and – if they encounter fertility problems – should have the same access to medical or surgical interventions (such as IVF) as detailed on pages 75–81. In the UK, there are some fairly complex legal implications to consider regarding donor insemination, though – mostly relating to parental rights and civil partnerships – about which more information can be found on websites listed in the Resources section from page 203.

1 in 6 adoptions in England in 2021 were to same-sex couples

If a trans person assigned female at birth (AFAB) is considering gender reassignment – with hormonal treatment and/or surgical transition – they may wish to preserve their

FEMALE HEALTH, FERTILITY & PREGNANCY

fertility beforehand. Egg harvesting (see page 81) would be
the usual option in these circumstances.

Adoption & foster caring

LGBTQ+ people have had the same rights to adopt a child
or become foster carers as other parents since 2005 in the
UK and the number of families with same-sex parents is
growing every year. Potential single parents should also not
be discriminated against if they wish to adopt or become a
foster carer either. This option can make a hugely valuable
contribution to your community, and change a child's life.

IMPORTANT!
Do not let other people pressure or coerce you into doing something against your will. It is your body, and your decision.

Choose the right option for you.

TESTING FOR PREGNANCY

You can buy a pregnancy test over-the-counter from your local pharmacy or supermarket, and they are also available at sexual health clinics. Most tests are more than 99 per cent accurate.

You can take a pregnancy test from the first day of a missed period. Doing one before that time isn't advisable since the level of the pregnancy hormone (human chorionic gonadotropin, or hCG) may be too low to show up on a test and might give a negative result even if you are pregnant. If you have an irregular cycle and are unsure about the timing of your period, the earliest time to take a test is three weeks after you've had unprotected sex.

Before you confirm things with a test, however, you may already have a suspicion that you're pregnant. A missed menstrual period is the most obvious sign, but other tell-tale symptoms can include tender, swollen breasts, a change in mood, and nausea (with or without vomiting).

Getting a positive pregnancy test result if you've planned a baby

Depending on your circumstances, receiving a positive pregnancy test may evoke a wide range of emotions. If you've planned to have a baby, you'll no doubt be walking on air and feeling hugely excited at this new chapter. As the reality sinks in, though, you may start to experience some less than positive feelings. A few of my patients worry they've made the wrong decision, and others become fearful about the act of giving birth. These are perfectly normal and natural responses, and there's no shame in discussing how you feel with your loved ones or a healthcare professional.

Once you've processed your good news, and are sure you want to go ahead with the pregnancy, you need to contact your healthcare provider to make a midwife assessment appointment (sometimes called the 'booking in' appointment). Here, you'll receive all the necessary antenatal advice, will be referred to your local hospital's maternity services, and will be listed for all the requisite scans and screenings. You'll receive a blood test at this appointment, too.

In reality, most GPs have little involvement with a person during their nine months of pregnancy, particularly if they are in good health with no associated complications. It's safer and more cost-effective for care to be offered by midwives, and nowadays, a pregnant person has a lot of autonomy and control in this important phase in their life. They'll be given

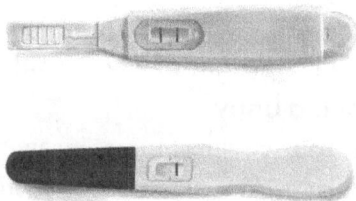

A positive pregnancy test will show two lines: control line and test line (see top test). A negative pregnancy test will just show the control line (see bottom test).

their own maternity health record, which will contain all the notes from the midwife, the family doctor, the hospital team, the sonographer and anyone else that might need to be involved (dietician, physiotherapist, social services, and so on). It is a really useful communication tool.

As a GP, I rarely have input in a patient's pregnancy, but will occasionally be contacted by a community midwife who may need specific advice or information, or by a consultant obstetrician if someone under their care requires prescribed medication. Other than that, the next time I see my patient they're often sitting in my surgery with a bouncing baby on their knee!

Getting a positive pregnancy test result if you've not planned a baby

If your positive pregnancy test is unexpected, you may feel lots of different emotions. Firstly, try not to panic; unexpected pregnancies can happen to any of us. Once you've got over the shock you will, of course, have to assess your options and decide how you wish to proceed. In order to help you with this, I'd urge you to talk things through with your partner, a trusted friend or family member, someone well placed to give you sensible, rational advice. But if you feel you can't talk to a loved one, you can book an appointment with your doctor or practice nurse, either of whom will treat you with care and sensitivity and will offer you informed and non-judgemental advice. There is also a wealth of advice available from charities and other organizations, too (see Resources from page 203).

Continuing with a pregnancy

Should you decide to go ahead with the pregnancy, the procedure on page 87 will apply. Some people may choose to continue with the pregnancy but have their baby adopted after the birth; this process would ordinarily be looked after by a local authority's social services department and/or an adoption agency.

Ending a pregnancy

If you live in England, Wales or Scotland and decide to terminate the pregnancy before 24 weeks, please make an appointment as soon as possible with your doctor, sexual health clinic or the British Pregnancy Advice Service (BPAS). A clinician will advise you and counsel you, without judgement or prejudice, and will refer you to an abortion clinic for further assessment and treatment. After 24 weeks, a termination can only be performed under extreme circumstances, for example if the mother's life is at risk or the child is likely to be born with severe disability.

You may also refer yourself to a private abortion clinic, where you'll have to pay for the procedure (the costs vary). Your local NHS sexual health clinic will have details of nearby services.

If you are under 16, your parents do not need to be told you are planning a termination, but you may be encouraged (but not pressured) to confide in a loved one for physical and mental support. Sometimes a family doctor will refer a patient to another colleague in the surgery if they are unable to participate in abortion for religious or ethical reasons.

Ending a pregnancy can be a traumatic experience that necessitates lots of help and support. See Resources from page 203 for organizations that offer advice and guidance.

The abortion law in Northern Ireland changed in March 2020. Women currently have access to a termination up until 12 weeks gestation (that is, 11 weeks and 6 days) without any conditions, and from 12 to 24 weeks if the pregnancy is impacting the woman's physical or mental health. Please consult the Resources section from page 203 for the most up-to-date guidelines.

EARLY PREGNANCY ISSUES

n general practice, if a patient experiences early pregnancy bleeding (about 20 per cent of women have some bleeding in the first 12 weeks of pregnancy) or any other associated complications, I immediately refer them to our local early pregnancy unit for an ultrasound scan. From that point on they'll be looked after by the midwife and the obstetrician who will update me on their condition. If the patient sadly suffers baby loss, I will contact them to offer my condolences and will signpost them for support (see Resources on page 203).

Miscarriage

Sadly, around one in every eight known pregnancies will end in miscarriage. Vaginal bleeding is the main sign, but light bleeding can be common in early pregnancy anyway. Always seek medical advice if you experience bleeding. Miscarriages can also occur without bleeding and are usually identified when your first pregnancy scan reveals the baby has no heartbeat. This is known as a missed miscarriage. After a miscarriage, the tissue of the pregnancy may pass out of your body naturally, or you may be given medicine or a surgical procedure to remove any remaining pregnancy tissue.

The majority of miscarriages occur in the first trimester. It is not usually possible to identify the exact cause, but miscarriages are rarely caused by something that you have done. It is believed that most early pregnancy loss is caused by abnormal chromosomes in the baby. Less commonly (one in four), miscarriages can occur in the second trimester.

A miscarriage can be extremely distressing. Look after yourself physically and emotionally. You will be referred to an early pregnancy unit and your doctor will be able to connect you with counselling services if you require them. And please remember that most miscarriages are one-off occurrences and can often be followed by a healthy pregnancy, if that is your wish.

Ectopic pregnancy

One in eighty women will suffer an ectopic pregnancy, when the fertilized egg (ovum) gets stuck somewhere outside the uterus. Common symptoms include:

- Acute or dull pain in the lower abdomen.
- Unusual vaginal bleeding.
- Feeling faint, or collapsing.
- Nausea and vomiting, or loss of appetite.
- Bowel or bladder problems.
- Breast pain.
- Delayed periods.
- Pain during sex.

An ectopic pregnancy is a medical emergency, so if you are pregnant and suspect this may be happening you must go to straight to A&E for urgent scanning and assessment.

Do not visit your family doctor, as this will only delay matters.

If you are experiencing these symptoms but have had a negative pregnancy test, particularly one that you think may be inaccurate – you must still flag this up to a clinician. Go straight to hospital. It could save your life.

Possible ectopic pregnancy sites

An ectopic pregnancy occurs when the fertilized egg (ovum) becomes stuck outside the uterus. This diagram highlights where an ectopic pregnancy can occur. On rare occasions, two pregnancies can occur that result in ectopic pregnancies. A heterotopic pregnancy is when two embryos are present in different places of the reproductive system and a twin ectopic pregnancy is when two embryos are stuck in the same place.

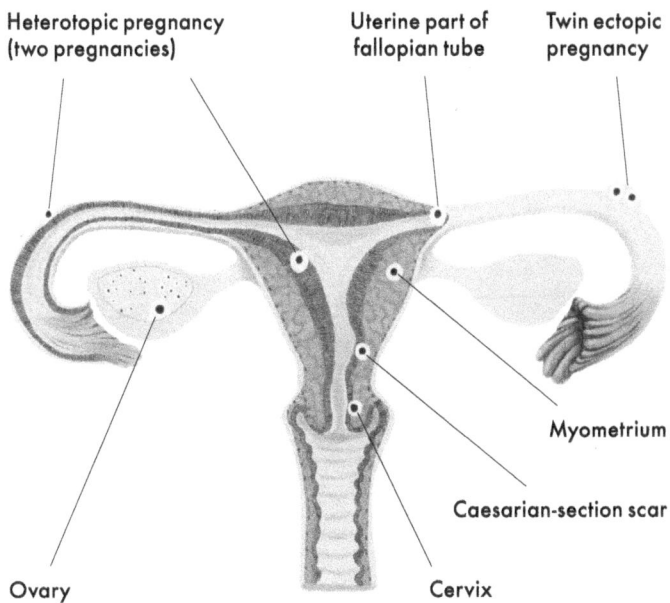

Heterotopic pregnancy
(two pregnancies)

Uterine part of
fallopian tube

Twin ectopic
pregnancy

Myometrium

Caesarian-section scar

Ovary

Cervix

YOUR BODY DURING PREGNANCY

Pregnancy is divided into three parts, know as trimesters, and during these trimesters your body is undertaking an incredible task – converting a bundle of cells into a living baby over a period of nine months (or 40 weeks). These months are not without their side effects, however, and many women can feel quite unwell at times during their pregnancy. The following pages are a guide to common pregnancy symptoms and those that warrant further attention from your doctor or pregnancy care team.

Many pregnant women find the first trimester particularly exhausting, something that is exacerbated by the fact that they often do not make their pregnancy public knowledge until after the first trimester is finished! The following areas of symptoms can be very common in pregnancy and shouldn't be cause for alarm. Please try to give yourself plenty of time to relax and acknowledge that you may need to take it easier over these next few months. As always, trust your instinct, and if you feel like any of these issues are particularly debilitating, then seek medical advice:

Common effects of pregnancy

- **Nausea & vomiting** is particularly common in the first trimester of pregnancy, but can ease off by weeks 16 to 20. Unfortunately, some women find they are nauseous all the way through pregnancy. Make sure you are drinking plenty of fluids and try eating small amounts more frequently, rather than eating large meals.

- **Heartburn & indigestion** are caused by hormonal changes and, in the later stages of pregnancy, by your baby pushing against your stomach. Eating little and often can help, as well as avoiding eating too close to bedtime and cutting down on spicy or rich foods. Over-the-counter heartburn medication is safe to use through pregnancy.

- **Bloating & constipation** are often caused by hormonal changes. Drink plenty of water, eat foods high in fibre, and try to keep some gentle exercise up to avoid too much discomfort.

- **Piles** can be common in pregnancy due to hormonal changes and can also be caused by constipation. They cause itching, soreness or swelling around your anus and occasional bleeding after you go to the toilet. Using the methods to avoid constipation (see above) and avoiding straining on the toilet can help. Holding a cold cloth over the area, or using moist toilet paper can ease discomfort.

- **Sensitive & swollen breasts** are again caused by hormonal changes as your body prepares for breastfeeding.

- **Leaking nipples** are common in the final weeks of pregnancy but can also occur months before your due date. As your body prepares for birth your breast tissue produces colostrum – a creamy, early milk – and this may leak out of your nipples before the baby is even born. Absorbent pads are available from pharmacies if required, or you could use good old-fashioned tissue inside your bra.

- **Thrush** (see *The Power of Puberty & Periods*) can be caused by the changing bacteria balance of your vagina during pregnancy. Over-the-counter treatments are available but you should consult your doctor or midwife before using these while you are pregnant.
- **Discharge** might increase in volume during pregnancy. Follow the advice in *The Power of Puberty & Periods* to determine if the colour of your discharge signals a problem.
- **Bleeding** during pregnancy can occur. It isn't always a problem, but you should always consult your doctor of midwife as it can be a sign of miscarriage (see page 93).

Other symptoms

- **Fatigue** is particularly noticeable in the first trimester, and many women are shocked by just how exhausted they feel. Unfortunately there is no solution to this other than to get as much rest as possible. Towards the later weeks of pregnancy you might find it difficult to sleep because your baby bump prevents you lying comfortably for long. You should try to sleep on your side in the last few months of pregnancy and may find using additional pillows under your bump as support can help you to be more comfortable.

- **Increased body temperature** is caused, again, by hormonal changes and an increased blood supply to the skin. Try to wear loose, comfortable clothing in natural fibres if possible.

- **Back pain** is caused in the early stage of pregnancy by your ligaments becoming softer and stretchier. Do not hesitate to speak to your doctor if it becomes extremely uncomfortable. Occasionally, back pain in your second or third trimesters could signify early labour, so consult your doctor or midwife if you are concerned.

- **Headaches** are another early pregnancy symptom that usually gets better as your pregnancy continues. Paracetamol is safe to take in pregnancy but consult your doctor if the headaches are severe, or if they are accompanied by signs of pre-eclampsia (see Hypertension, page 105).

- **Teeth and gums** are susceptible to plaque during pregnancy if you do not follow good oral hygiene. For this reason, in the UK, NHS dental care is free to expectant mothers during pregnancy and in the first year of their baby's life. If you are suffering with vomiting (see page 99) then try to rinse your mouth with water after you have vomited to reduce acid attacking your teeth.

- **Taste and smell** can change during your pregnancy with some women experiencing an unpleasant metallic or bitter taste throughout their pregnancy, or experiencing either a loss of smell, reduced smell or noticing a persistent strong smell. (I went through this, smelling petrol and coffee wherever I went, throughout my pregnancies.)

- **Nosebleeds, a blocked nose and nasal ulcers** are other unfortunate side effects of pregnancy, caused by those hormonal changes again!

- **Pelvic pain** can be felt across the front and back of your pelvis, as well as over your perineum during pregnancy. The pain can be lessened and managed by introducing specialist exercises to strengthen the area or using a pelvic support belt. Consult your doctor or midwife for a referral to a physiotherapist.

- **Stretch marks** are very common in pregnancy and caused by stretching of the skin as your bump grows, along with hormonal changes that make skin more susceptible to stretch marks. They look like pink, red, purple or brown streaks (depending on your skin colour) and may feel itchy. Those susceptible to keloid scars may find they have more pronounced stretch marks. Although they may fade after the baby is born, they are unlikely to disappear completely. There's little evidence that beauty creams can prevent stretch marks, but keeping the skin moisturized might help ease any discomfort.

Pregnancy can feel like a complete mess of unwanted side effects, but remember it doesn't last forever!

- **Swollen ankles, fingers and feet** are caused by your body holding more water than usual when you are pregnant, and the extra water gathers on the lower parts of your body if you have been standing for long periods. Try to rest with your feet up wherever possible and keep up regular, gentle exercise. Gradual swelling is normal and not harmful but a sudden increase is sometimes a sign of pre-eclampsia (see Hypertension, page 105).
- **Weight gain** is caused not only by your growing baby and placenta but also by fat stores laid down to prepare your body for breastfeeding. Weight gain varies dramatically between women but most fall within the 10–12.5kg range. Try to stick to a healthy diet and gentle exercise during pregnancy. If you are worried about weight gain, do not embark on a weight-loss diet without consulting your doctor.

Pregnancy complications

Some conditions brought on by pregnancy will require more medical attention, so alert your doctor or midwife if you experience the following:

- **Severe vomiting**, also known as hyperemesis gravidarum, is defined as vomitting many times a day and being unable to keep food and drink down. This poses a risk that you will become dehydrated and may require hospital treatment.

- **Deep vein thrombosis (DVT)** is the occurrence of a blood clot in one of the veins deep in your body and can have serious consequences. Your risk of DVT is slightly increased by pregnancy and you will be more at risk if you have an existing condition that makes clots more likely, are over 35 years old, have a family history of blood clots, smoke or are obese.
- **Gestational diabetes** is when your body cannot produce enough insulin during pregnancy and will usually be detected at a routine antenatal blood sugar screening. Your pregnancy will be closely managed and you will be given advice on controlling your blood sugar levels. It will usually go away after you have given birth.
- **Hypertension, or high blood pressure**, can be detected during routine antenatal blood pressure checks and you will be advised on how to manage it. If you have hypertension during pregnancy you are also at greater risk of pre-eclampsia, a condition in the placenta in later pregnancy, that needs to be closely monitored by your doctor.
- **Intrahepatic cholestasis** of pregnancy is a liver condition in which bile from the liver builds up in your body. Its main symptom is itching without a rash (although harmless itching is also common in pregnancy, see Stretch marks, page 103) and you'll be offered regular liver function tests, as it can potentially have serious consequences for your baby.

ANTENATAL MENTAL HEALTH

I t's not unusual for women to struggle with their mental health during this pivotal time in their lives. Indeed, some may develop emotional and psychological issues for the first time during the perinatal phase, perhaps experiencing feelings they've never had before. Not only can your mood and behaviour be affected by the fluctuation of your hormones, you may naturally find yourself becoming very anxious about your unborn baby, for instance, or worrying about your future parenting skills. If these feelings become overwhelming, please don't suffer in silence; instead, speak with a healthcare professional who will assess your symptoms and signpost you to the relevant resources. You might be referred for some talking therapy, or you may be advised to join a local antenatal group where you get together with other mums-to-be.

I'm a huge advocate of self-care, too. Pregnancy can be tough, both physically and emotionally, and you shouldn't feel guilty about giving yourself some serious tender loving care.

If you already suffer with any underlying mental health conditions – such as psychosis or bipolar disorder – you should always flag these up with your doctor or midwife, who'll ensure you receive the appropriate support and monitoring with input from the obstetrics and gynaecology department.

Also, please be aware that if you're on anti-depressants and become pregnant, or are looking to conceive, there is no need to stop your medication. It is now thought that most women are safe to continue their SSRI anti-depressants throughout their pregnancy. Talk things through with your doctor, who may suggest a referral to an obstetrics and gynaecology consultant with a specialism in maternal mental health, and/or the setting up of a joint care arrangement with your psychiatrist. In addition, there are some great charities out there that offer lots of support and guidance for potential parents to care for their mental health (see Resources from page 203 for more information).

Pregnancy TLC

Write down your thoughts in a mood diary (this can help to process your feelings).

Have a nice catch-up with a good friend, colleague or neighbour over a cup of coffee.

Give yourself half an hour to put your feet up and watch television, read a book, listen to a podcast or anything that gives you a bit of 'me time'.

PREGNANCY IN BLACK, ASIAN & ETHNIC
MINORITY COMMUNITIES

can't cover the subject of pregnancy without touching on a topic that continues to shock and sadden me. Statistics from the MBRRACE-UK group (Mothers and babies: Reducing risk through audits and confidential enquiries across the UK) show that Black women are *four* times more likely to die in pregnancy and childbirth than white women. Mixed ethnicity and Asian women are *twice* as likely to suffer this fate. And elsewhere there's a similar picture: the World Health Organization recognizes that Black and Asian women have poorer outcomes in pregnancy and post-natal care.

There can be no doubt about it: these women have been failed by the healthcare system. For decades, issues around perinatal pain (pain in pregnancy) have not been taken as seriously in Black and ethnic minority women, and birth complications haven't been picked up soon enough. This issue has been overlooked and neglected for far too long, but I'm encouraged that work is now being done to address this inequality at an institutional level, via the Department of Health and Social Care's Women's Health Strategy and the Royal College of Obstetricians and Gynaecologist's *Better for Women* report. An all-party Parliamentary group on Black maternal health has been established and, every September, Black Maternal Health Week takes place aimed at raising awareness and tackling institutionalized racism in the healthcare system.

The fundamental point is that the colour of a woman's skin should *not* impact upon her pregnancy and childbirth experience. If you believe you are not receiving the healthcare you deserve, and are not being listened to or treated with respect, you *must* flag up your concerns and make a complaint (see Resources from page 203 for organizations offering help and support). Sadly, while these inequalities persist, if you are from an ethnic minority, it becomes even more important that you are aware of your health and monitor any changes yourself (see pages 19–23 and 31–35 for advice on self examination).

Black women in the UK are 4 times more likely to die in pregnancy and childbirth than white women

CHILDBIRTH

The excitement builds as you near the end of your pregnancy, and you will have your midwife or doctor to guide you through the birth itself.

As you approach the later stages of pregnancy, you may want to write a birth plan. A birth plan outlines your ideal birth but it may need to be adjusted as the actual situation unfolds.

A birth plan may include subjects like:

- Pain relief during labour.
- Delivery positions.
- Assisted delivery preferences (forceps or a ventouse suction cup, if required during the birth).
- Location, including home, birth centre or hospital, and other preferences, such as water births.
- Timeline for holding the baby.
- Having your partner cut the umbilical cord.

You also need to decide who will be present at the birth. Some couples employ the services of a doula, a layperson who is trained as a labour companion. Doulas aren't medical professionals; their primary role is to offer emotional and physical support during labour. Doulas can be involved throughout an entire pregnancy or just for labour and delivery. They can also offer support and advice after the birth (post-partum). Talk with your partner and decide who you want to have attending the birth. Some couples feel that this is a private time and prefer not to have others present.

Breech & transverse babies

Your baby's position inside the uterus will be checked at your pregnancy appointments. Most babies naturally turn into a head-down position towards the end of pregnancy but sometimes they will still be feet-down (breech) or lying sideways (transverse) beyond 36 weeks of pregnancy. If this is the case then your healthcare provider will discuss your options, which can include an external cephalic version, a process in which a healthcare professional will try to reposition the baby by applying pressure on your abdomen. This successfully repositions around half of breech babies but, if the baby cannot be repositioned into a head-down position, then your doctor will discuss your childbirth options, including viability of a vaginal birth or the option of a Caesarean section delivery.

The process of childbirth

Of course every labour and birth is different, but these are the stages you will go through on your journey to parenthood.

Amniotic sac rupture

During pregnancy, your baby sits in a fluid-filled membrane called the amniotic sac. This sac will rupture, usually before you go into labour or at the start of labour, and is commonly referred to as your 'waters breaking'. It can either feel like a gentle trickle or a sudden gush of fluid, and the fluid should be clear and odourless. When your waters break, contact the labour ward, midwife, obstetrician or other obstetric care provider and follow their guidance. Occasionally, the amniotic sac can stay intact throughout labour and the baby delivered inside the sac. Your midwife or doctor may advise that your waters are broken manually (referred to as 'artificial rupture of membranes') as the rupture of the amniotic sac can release hormones that are thought to help with labour.

Contractions
For the baby to move through the cervix your uterine muscles will repeatedly tighten and release in a motion known as contractions. They can feel like strong period cramps or a tight internal pressure that begins in your back and moves towards the front. Contractions are likely to occur throughout labour and come closer together as you approach active labour (although their frequency can ebb and flow). A minute-long contraction, repeating itself at least five minutes apart, for an hour, is generally seen as a reliable indication that you are in active labour.

Many pregnant women will also experience contractions intermittently in their second or third trimesters, when they are not in labour. These are referred to as Braxton-Hicks contractions and mean that contractions aren't always a reliable indicator of labour.

Stage 1: Dilation of the cervix

This first stage of active labour (and childbirth) is considered to be when your cervix has dilated 4cm or more. The cervix is a tubular structure approximately 3–4cm in length with a passage that connects the uterine cavity to the vagina. Its purpose is to keep the uterus closed through pregnancy, and then, when labour begins, it will dilate (open up) to allow the baby to be born. In the final weeks of your pregnancy, hormonal changes will cause your cervical tissue to soften and get thinner, which enables it to open more easily during labour. The cervical canal will continue opening up until it has reached 10cm in diameter and the baby is able to pass into the birth canal.

Stage 2: The birth

Once your cervix is fully dilated to 10cm, the baby will pass through the birth canal. At this point, the skin and muscles around your vagina, labia and perineum will stretch, and you may feel a burning sensation (sometimes referred to as 'the ring of fire') when they reach their maximum stretching capacity.

Your skin and muscles may tear to allow the baby through, they may be able to stretch sufficiently on their own, or your doctor or midwife may decide to perform an episiotomy by making a small cut to the vagina to enlarge the opening. Tears and cuts can be common, particularly in a first birth, and will usually be repaired with dissolvable stitches after the placenta has been delivered.

The downwards pressure of the baby passing through

your birth canal will ease as their head emerges from the vagina. The baby might need a bit of help from your midwife or doctor to clear the amniotic fluid from its lungs or its first cries might naturally clear them.

Usually, the baby's shoulders will be delivered in the next push or contraction and the midwife or doctor may rotate the baby's head slightly to make the passage of the shoulders a little easier. Once the shoulders have passed out of the vagina, the feet will easily slip out and you have delivered your baby!

Stage 3: Delivery of the placenta

The placenta and the amniotic sac that supported and protected the baby during pregnancy will still be in the uterus after the delivery. These need to be delivered, which can happen straight away or may take a little time. Your midwife or doctor can help speed along delivery of the placenta by massaging your abdomen or offering an injection of syntometrine or syntocinon medication to stimulate its release. Delivering the placenta can cause further feelings of pressure in your uterus (although not as strong as the pressure during the birth), and you may need to push to move it through the birth canal. Your midwife or doctor will then check to ensure that all of the placenta has been safely delivered.

After delivery of the placenta, you may have an examination to determine if stitches are needed to help heal any cuts or tears from labour. Smaller cuts and tears will often heal of their own accord but the doctor may repair larger ones with stitches, that will dissolve as the body heals.

Stage 1: Dilation of the cervix

The cervix dilates to allow your baby to pass through. Once the cervix has dilated 4cm you are considered to be in active labour and it will continue dilating up to 10cm when your baby can pass through.

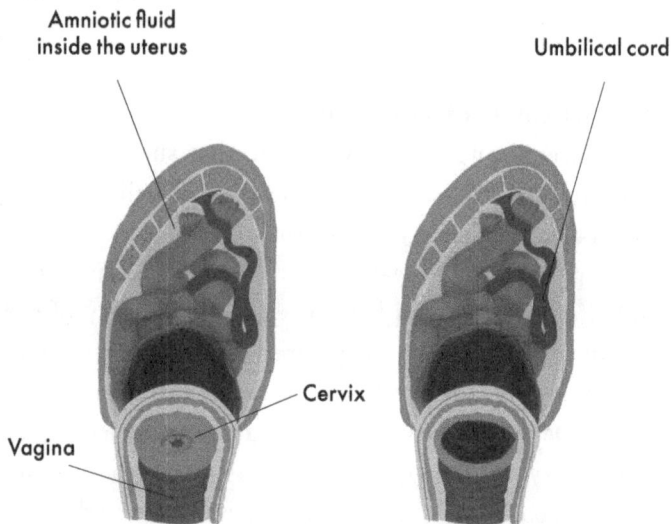

Amniotic fluid
inside the uterus

Umbilical cord

Cervix

Vagina

1 Before active labour, the undilated cervix is closed to safely hold your baby inside the uterus.

2 A fully dilated cervix is 10cm or more in diameter, large enough to allow the baby to pass through ready for Stage 2, the birth.

Stage 2: The birth

Once the cervix is fully dilated, your contractions will push the baby through the vaginal canal to be born. This stage of labour, often called the 'pushing stage', can be very hard work and you may feel an overwhelming urge to push to aid the baby on its journey.

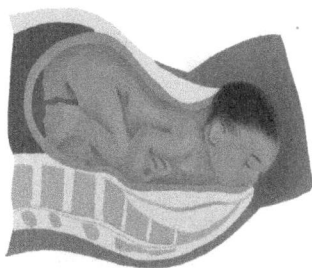

1 Presentation of the head as the baby passes through the vagina (birth canal) and the head emerges from the vulva.

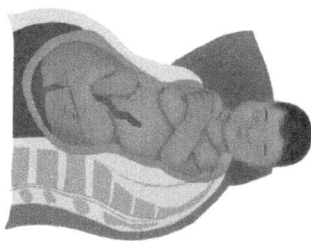

2 Rotation and delivery of anterior shoulder will usually occur in the next contraction after the head has emerged.

Placenta

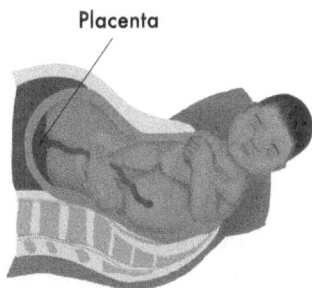

3 Once one shoulder has emerged the baby's position will move slightly to enable the other shoulder to be released.

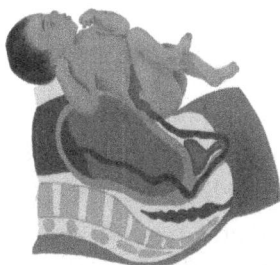

4 The rest of the body will swiftly follow, with the umbilical cord remaining attached to the baby.

Stage 3: Delivery of the placenta

It is important to ensure that the whole placenta, amniotic sac and umbilical cord are removed from the uterus after the birth. This can happen naturally or you can be given treatment to speed up delivery.

Detached placenta   Umbilical cord

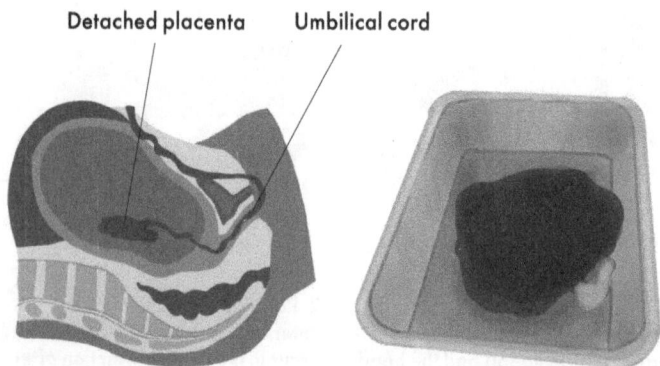

1 The placenta detaches from the uterus and exits through the vagina.

2 The placenta will be checked by your doctor or midwife to ensure it is complete.

The moments after giving birth

The time immediately after you have given birth is very special but the experience differs significantly for different mothers. You will probably be completely exhausted or still be feeling the effects of painkilling drugs, so be gentle with yourself. Your midwife or doctor will do a check of the baby's health and, all being well, you or your partner will be given the baby to hold. Many new parents like to enjoy 'skin-to-skin' time in the first moments after the birth, where your baby's bare skin is in direct contact with your skin. This is believed to help the baby to establish breastfeeding (if that is how you choose to feed your baby) and encourage bonding. Dads and non-birthing partners can benefit from skin-to-skin contact too so it's a wonderful time to enjoy some special moments with your new family.

The practice of placentophagy (consuming your placenta either cooked or dehydrated into capsule form) is gaining recognition as advocates believe it can help boost post-birth recovery, but there isn't any firm evidence of this.

If you gave birth in a hospital or a midwife-led unit, the length of time that you spend there after giving birth will depend on your circumstances and the baby's health, but you should be given an option to discuss how you'd like to feed the baby.

POST-NATAL ISSUES

While many post-natal conditions are addressed directly by midwives and health visitors, I will often see new mums in my surgery who have been referred to me for prescription medication to treat a variety of issues.

Physical issues
Your body has been through a lot during pregnancy and birth, and you may experience a few of the following issues afterwards.

Post-partum bleeding
It is common to experience some bleeding, known as lochia, for two to six weeks after birth. You should not use any internal period products (such as tampons or menstrual cups) for the first six weeks after giving birth as it could increase your chance of getting an infection. Most women will use sanitary towels, which should be changed regularly. It's also a good idea to bathe or shower daily to keep your genitals clean as they heal.

Painful breastfeeding & mastitis
Midwives and health visitors usually work with mums to manage any breastfeeding issues in their specialized assisting clinics. However, if you are suffering with mastitis – a painful

inflammation of breast tissue usually resulting from an infection – you may be referred to your family doctor to be prescribed appropriate antibiotics. The hormones released during breastfeeding can also cause vaginal atrophy (see *The Power of Menopause & Midlife*). In the first few days after birth some women also find that breastfeeding causes extreme cramps in the uterus as hormonal changes prompt the uterus to contract down to its pre-pregnancy size.

Post-partum infections

If you are suffering with uterine, bladder or kidney infections following childbirth, you may need to be prescribed a course of antibiotics.

Haemorrhoids & constipation

The pushing and straining of labour, and nine months of raised abdominal pressure, can cause haemorrhoids and constipation. In order to minimize these uncomfortable conditions, your doctor might advise you to follow a high-fibre diet, drink lots of water and perhaps take laxatives.

Post-natal vaginal discharge

A thin, white, odourless vaginal discharge is normal. However, refer to *The Power of Puberty & Periods* for tips on when a review with your doctor may be necessary.

Post-natal incontinence

Urge and stress incontinence is common during and after pregnancy, which is why it's always a good idea to maintain a healthy weight before you decide to have a baby. Pelvic floor exercises (see *The Power of Menopause & Midlife*) can help to tighten your muscles – and incontinence pads can make you feel more comfortable – but if you're leaking a lot of urine, don't put up with it. If it's affecting your quality of life, speak to your doctor who may be able to refer you for a scan and some urodynamic studies (tests of the lower urinary tract).

Wellbeing after childbirth

The first year with a new baby can be a challenge. I want you to be aware of how to look after your own wellbeing and know when to ask for help.

Post-natal depression

This mood variation can affect parents after having a baby. Symptoms include: constant sadness, difficulty bonding, lack of energy, irritability, feelings of guilt and inadequacy. New mums often experience 'baby blues' but this is short term, whereas post-natal depression is longer, more persistent and with more intrusive thoughts. It can affect both birth and non-birth parents.

Post-partum psychosis

This affects 1 in 500 women in the UK and must be treated as a medical emergency. Symptoms are severe and usually start within the first two days, often within hours, of giving birth (although it can also develop several weeks later). Symptoms can be similar to post-natal depression but also include extreme confusion, delusions, hallucinations, paranoia and suicidal thoughts and actions, making it the leading cause of maternal death in the UK. It is under-researched, and there is a particular lack of awareness in Black and Asian communities, but the condition must be quickly assessed, treated and monitored by perinatal mental health services, as recovery is possible.

Post-natal sex

Whenever you're ready as a couple, both in mind and body, you can start to have sex again. The emotional rollercoaster of childbirth can have a real impact on your sex life – think perineal trauma, Caesarean section scar, breastfeeding pain and sleep deprivation – so take your time, do not be pressured and seek support if needed. And be aware it is possible to become pregnant again immediately (see below).

Post-natal contraception

If you're not breastfeeding, you can use your usual contraception (see *The Power of Puberty & Periods*). If you are breastfeeding, the IUD, barrier methods, or progesterone-only contraceptives (the POP, IUS, or contraceptive implant or injection) are recommended. It is not true that you can't get pregnant if you have just had a baby, are breastfeeding or aren't menstruating. You can!

Post-natal menstruation

If you are not breastfeeding, periods typically return 6–12 weeks after you give birth. If you are breastfeeding, this can vary because the hormone that prompts you to make milk can prevent your body making the hormones that control menstruation so you might not bleed at all. Your periods may only resume when you stop breastfeeding completely. If your periods haven't returned within 12 months of stopping breastfeeding, see your doctor.

Planning for another baby

Although women may be able to get pregnant just a few weeks after giving birth, this is not always safe for them or their babies. Ideally pregnancies should be spaced 18–24 months apart. This will give your body time to replenish its nutrients, heal inflammation and repair any organ damage. Getting pregnant too soon (or leaving too long between pregnancies) can result in premature birth, pre-eclampsia or placental abruption.

GYNAECOLOGICAL AREAS OF CONCERN

There are a number of conditions and syndromes that can adversely affect women's health during their fertile years, but often their suffering is not investigated until they find they do not conceive as quickly as hoped. Even if you are not planning on starting a family now, or ever, I urge you to read these pages as the conditions can affect anyone, so awareness of them is vital to receiving the healthcare you deserve.

Polycystic ovary syndrome

Polycystic ovary syndrome (PCOS) is a very common condition that affects about one in five post-pubescent women, although over half of them don't notice any symptoms. PCOS is a lifelong metabolic, hormonal imbalance condition associated with high levels of insulin (a hormone made by the pancreas that regulates blood sugar levels), that can lead to an over-production which, in turn, affects the normal ovulation process. The development of chronic health issues, such as high cholesterol and type 2 diabetes, in later life has also been associated with having PCOS, as have psychological diagnoses such as depression and anxiety. It also seems to run in families, so you may be more at risk if your female relatives have been affected by the condition. Symptoms can often be more severe if you're obese or overweight.

Many women are given their diagnosis in their late teens and early twenties, although it can also be flagged up later when they're having problems getting pregnant. They might start monitoring their menstrual cycle and realize they have irregular periods (or no periods at all) and, as a result of haphazard or absent ovulation, they often find it difficult to conceive.

The biggest worry many women have when given a diagnosis of polycystic ovaries or polycystic ovary syndrome is that they'll have difficulty becoming pregnant. However, from my clinical experience, if the person is below the age of 35, has a healthy weight and diet and also takes clomifene citrate (clomid) or metformin (see page 77), they have a 70–80 per cent chance of becoming pregnant.

Symptoms of PCOS
- Irregular or absent menstrual periods, which are caused by your ovaries not regularly releasing an egg.
- Excess hair (hirsutism) on your face, back, chest or buttocks, or thinning hair on the head, which is caused by excessive levels of androgen (a male hormone). This can also cause weight gain and oily skin or bad acne.
- Polycystic ovaries, which occur when your ovaries become enlarged, and multiple follicles (fluid-filled sacs) can develop. These sacs surround the egg and may prevent it from being released.

Diagnosis of PCOS

To be diagnosed with PCOS, you need to present with at least two of the above symptoms. Despite the name of the condition, you don't actually need to have cysts in your ovaries as a qualifying factor; you could just have the irregular periods and excess androgen. Conversely and confusingly, you can also have polycystic ovaries without having the syndrome; some women may possess a large number of harmless follicles in their ovaries (up to 8mm in size), but don't present with irregular periods and/or excess androgen.

Polycystic ovaries

Confusingly, you can have polycystic ovaries without having PCOS, and some women can have effects of PCOS (excessive androgen and irregular periods) without having cysts on their ovaries (see page 128 for more details). The opposite diagram shows a polycystic ovary next to a healthy ovary. In the healthy ovary, one follicle will mature to release an egg at ovulation each month, but in the polycystic ovary the cysts on the ovary are swollen and sore. Because there are a number of cysts, the follicles can be prevented from maturing so no egg is released and ovulation does not occur.

Healthy ovary

Ovary with PCOS

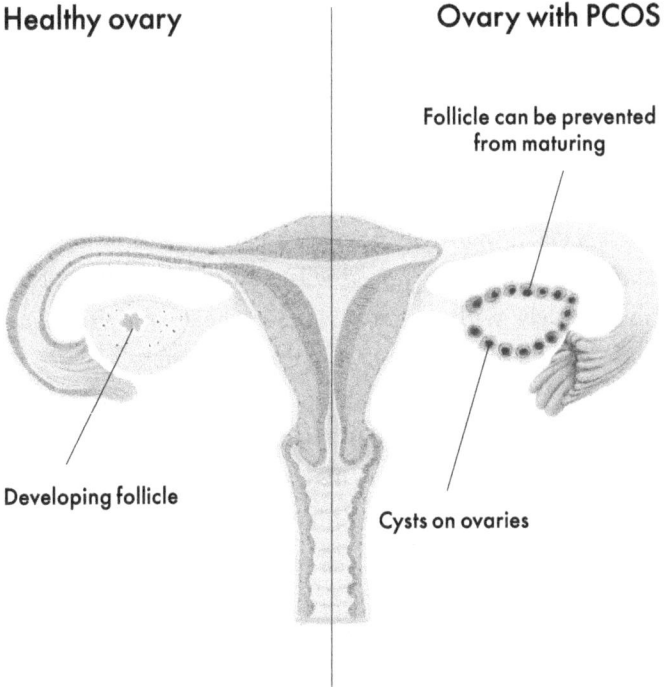

Follicle can be prevented from maturing

Developing follicle

Cysts on ovaries

Treatment of PCOS

There is no cure for PCOS, but it can be managed. Treatment is more often than not based around individual symptoms, for example a person with a high BMI might embark on a weight-loss programme, usually incorporating a healthy, balanced diet. Someone with insulin resistance may receive similar advice, but may also be prescribed the drug metformin, which is commonly used to treat people with type 2 diabetes.

A patient with menstrual irregularities can take the combined or progesterone-only contraceptive pill or, if they prefer, can be fitted with an IUS coil (see *The Power of Puberty & Periods*). Excessive hair growth on the face and body can be addressed with ruby laser treatment or, alternatively, with a topical eflornithine cream or an anti-androgen medication (such as spironolactone).

An individual with severe acne can often respond well to a medication called Dianette (which also has contraceptive properties) because it has high levels of anti-androgens. However these benefits will have to be weighed up for a person with a BMI of over 30, because of the increased risk of blood clots.

Once diagnosed with PCOS, you should be monitored for early signs of health problems. This may involve the following:

- **Regular blood pressure checks** which you can do at home before discussing the readings with your doctor. Blood pressure monitors can be purchased easily, and you may find it useful to keep a diary of the readings; there's a great one to download and print from the British Hypertension Society (see Resources from page 203).

- **Diabetes checks** will be undertaken depending on your weight, lifestyle, BMI and family history. You may be entitled to an HbA1c diabetes blood test and a fasting cholesterol test every one to three years.
- **Checks for cancer of the uterus** should ideally be undertaken every three to four months to check for any thickening of the lining of the uterus and to therefore reduce the chances of uterine cancer. If you've not had a period for four months and you're not on contraceptives to stop your periods, talk to your doctor. They may be able to give you a medication such as a contraceptive to regulate your period, or might send you for an ultrasound scan to check the lining of the uterus.

Living with PCOS

If you feel PCOS has affected your mood or has caused depression, you can either bring it up with your doctor or self-refer to your local Healthy Minds service (usually contactable via your local NHS foundation trust website) where you may benefit from talking therapy.

Women with PCOS tend to reach menopause about two years later than the average but symptoms of PCOS do not disappear with menopause. Testosterone levels will decrease in post-menopause but from a higher point than

FEMALE HEALTH, FERTILITY & PREGNANCY

in women without PCOS. Small studies have found that testosterone levels in post-menopausal women are roughly equal, in those with and without PCOS, about 20 years after menopause.

Adenomyosis

Adenomyosis is a little-known (and much misdiagnosed) condition that sees the inner lining of the uterus (endometrium) breaking into the muscle wall of the uterus (myometrium), causing inflammation, thickening and stiffening.

Like endometriosis (see page 140), this is not an infection, it's not contagious, and it's a benign (not cancerous) condition. Nobody is quite sure why it occurs, but it's likely that most sufferers will have a genetic predisposition to it. About one-third of women with adenomyosis experience few or no symptoms whatsoever; it's often picked up by chance during an ultrasound scan checking for another condition.

Adenomyosis may be less recognizable than endometriosis, but it still affects a significant number of people; it's thought that one in ten women have it, more commonly women in their forties and fifties who have had children. That said, in my clinical practice I've seen many patients in their twenties and thirties who present to me with pelvic pain and heavy periods, who are eventually diagnosed with adenomyosis. Very sadly, some have suffered miscarriages. Maintaining a pregnancy can be more difficult if the uterus lining is stiffened and the uterus is prevented from expanding, so anyone with adenomyosis may be at higher risk of losing their baby or having a premature birth. They may require close monitoring from a specialist consultant.

Research on this is scant, but it's thought that adenomyosis is unlikely to hinder conception and fertility. Unlike endometriosis, it doesn't usually cause scarring to the fallopian tubes and ovaries, which can hinder eggs from travelling towards sperm for fertilization.

Symptoms of adenomyosis

- Severe menstrual cramps.
- Heavy or painful periods and irregular periods.
- Irregular periods.
- Pelvic pain.
- Pressure or discomfort in the lower abdomen.
- Bloating before your period.
- Pain during or after sex.
- Severe anaemia (due to heavy periods).

Diagnosis of adenomyosis

It can take many years to diagnose adenomyosis. Being such an obscure and unrecognized condition, it often gets missed or misdiagnosed as severe period pain (dysmenorrhea) or uterine fibroids (see page 152) and, in some cases, is confused with endometriosis. A transvaginal ultrasound scan of the pelvis can assist with the diagnosis, but this tends to happen only when the condition is in its advanced stages, when the uterine walls have become extremely thickened, and by which time the patient may have suffered horrendously for years. Other than this, the condition is detected by a laparoscopy (see page 150) or an MRI scan.

Treatment of adenomyosis

As with endometriosis, there is no cure for adenomyosis, but we as family doctors can help to manage a patient's pain and discomfort. For those at the milder end of the pain spectrum, a combination of painkillers and hormonal contraceptives can help to keep symptoms at bay, as can the addition of some lifestyle changes (diet, exercise, and so on).

I'll usually discuss the following treatment pathways with my adenomyosis patients in order to ascertain what best suits their needs (most of the options are similar to those offered for endometriosis). As always with women's health, there's rarely a one-size-fits-all solution.

- **Pain relief** (paracetamol and/or ibuprofen, if the latter can be tolerated).
- **Hormone regulation treatment** (for example, oral contraceptive pill, implant, injection or IUS coil).
- **Mefenamic acid**, which can help with pain and bleeding, if tolerated.
- **Tranexamic acid**, a medication prescribed for heavy periods that can reduce pain and bleeding.
- **Ablation,** a surgical procedure that involves burning away a layer on the inside of the uterus, which can reduce or eliminate heavy bleeding.
- **Hysterectomy,** the surgical removal of the uterus, can be an option for severe cases of adenomyosis.

Hysterectomy is the only sure-fire way of permanently ridding yourself of severe adenomyosis. This is often a viable treatment for older women, but is not always preferable for young, fertile women who aim to get pregnant one day. Sadly, family doctors such as myself often find themselves having very frank conversations with patients who are desperate to rid themselves of the pain and suffering associated with adenomyosis (and endometriosis), but who are still keen to have babies; it's a heart-rending dilemma to face. There is a little piece of light at the end of the tunnel, though; adenomyosis symptoms tend to improve as women in their forties and fifties transition into the menopause.

Effects of adenomyosis

The endometrium is the lining of the uterus that thickens and breaks away during a menstrual cycle; it is encased in a muscle wall called the myometrium. Adenomyosis is a condition that sees the endometrium lining breaking into and embedding itself into the myometrium. This causes the myometrium to thicken and can result in feelings of pain, pressure and bloating, severe menstrual cramps, heavy and irregular periods, anaemia or pain during sex.

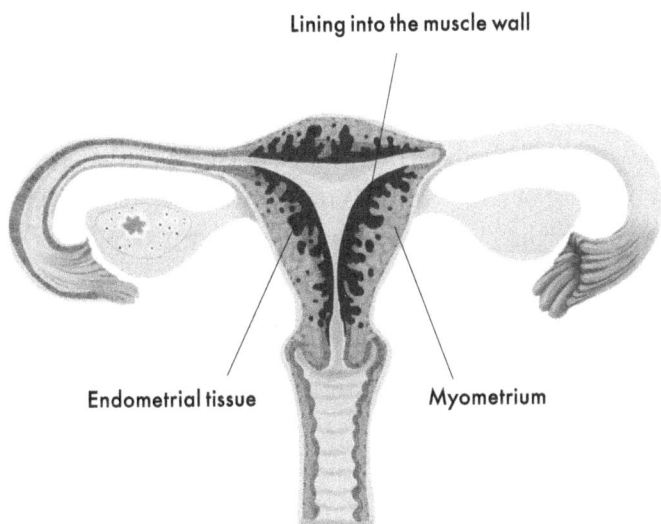

Lining into the muscle wall

Endometrial tissue

Myometrium

Living with adenomyosis

The painful symptoms associated with adenomyosis, especially if it left untreated, can detrimentally affect your physical and emotional wellbeing. If the heavy periods and pelvic pain aren't bad enough to contend with, there's also a debilitating and uncomfortable condition called 'adenomyosis belly'. This is caused when the uterine walls grow and thicken, putting pressure on surrounding organs like the bladder and intestine. This in turn leads to a bloated, protruding abdomen which, for obvious reasons, can have a terrible effect on someone's self-confidence. I know a lot of women who've been told by their doctors that they've got a bad case of IBS (irritable bowel syndrome), or have just put on weight, but who've then gone on to get a diagnosis of adenomyosis. This is the reason why we desperately need to increase research and awareness!

> You can have PCOS, adenomyosis and endometriosis all together.

Endometriosis

Endometriosis is an inflammatory lifelong, systemic condition that occurs when microscopic cells similar to those found in the lining of the uterus – known as the endometrium – are distributed around the pelvis, abdomen and, sometimes, other areas of the body. During a woman's menstrual cycle, these cells behave in the same way as those in the uterus by building up and breaking down. However, unlike the cells of the uterus – which are evacuated from the body as a period – this endometrial tissue has no way of escaping. It instead grows outside the uterus, spreading adhesions and causing inflammation irrespective of if you are having a period and remaining attached to different areas of the body. This may include:

- The ovaries and the fallopian tubes.
- The outer side of the uterus.
- The lining of the inside of the abdomen.
- The bowel or bladder.

These growths can cause severe pain and inflammation, and can sometimes lead to scarring (also known as fibrous adhesions). As the fibrous adhesions progressively grow, the inflammatory response to the growths can cause all-over body pain and fatigue.

In the UK, it is estimated that one in ten women are living with endometriosis (although data from the Australian Institute of Health and Welfare suggests it's as many as one in seven females). It's a condition that can affect you from your teenage years to your midlife years. Most sufferers are diagnosed between the ages of 25 and 40 – although, for many, the impact can have lasting repercussions. It is thought that the condition may be passed through the genes, so if your mum or an aunt has the condition, you may well be more susceptible. Having dealt with numerous cases of endometriosis in my surgery, I know just how distressing and debilitating it can be.

Symptoms of endometriosis

- Painful or heavy periods (with or without clots).
- Pain during or after sex (particularly if penetration is deep).
- Pain during ovulation.
- Painful bowel movements.
- Sharp or burning pain during or following a bowel movement, that's especially prevalent during your period.
- Pain when passing urine.
- Leg pain and cramps.
- Back pain.
- Bowel and bladder pain, in some cases due to endometrial adhesions.
- Diarrhoea, constipation and bloating.
- Fatigue and lack of energy.
- Infertility.
- Depression.

Diagnosis of endometriosis

On average, it takes about seven years – yes, you read that correctly, *seven years* – for a woman to receive a confirmed endometriosis diagnosis. This is often the case because its signs and symptoms can be mistaken for other conditions like heavy periods. The diagnostic process will start with your doctor who, after obtaining a full medical history from you, may carry out an internal pelvic examination or recommend an ultrasound scan to detect ovarian cysts or scar tissue that may have been caused by endometriosis. It's not always straightforward, however, because an ultrasound scan can be reported as normal and yet the patient can have endometriosis. Some patients are referred to a gynaecologist for a laparoscopy, a minor operation performed under general anaesthetic in which a camera is inserted into the pelvis. Endometriosis can only be confirmed with this surgical examination; the consultant will take a biopsy that will be examined very carefully to look for signs of the condition. This is currently the gold-standard method of diagnosing endometriosis.

Infuriatingly, far too many women are suffering needlessly with endometriosis because they haven't been taken seriously enough by a clinician. Do not let anyone normalize or trivialize your pain and, ideally, back up your case and empower yourself with personal data from a tracker app (or a diary) on which you record your symptoms each month. Monitoring how painful or heavy your periods are will make it easier for you and your doctor to see if there are any patterns emerging. If you still feel you're not being listened to, you have the right to change your doctor, preferably to one with a special interest in women's health.

Effects of endometriosis

The endometrium is the lining of the uterus that thickens and breaks away during a menstrual cycle. Endometriosis refers to a condition in which tiny cells, similar to those of the endometrial lining, break away from their usual position and embed themselves in other areas of the abdomen. The diagram opposite shows some of the places where these cells can situate themselves.

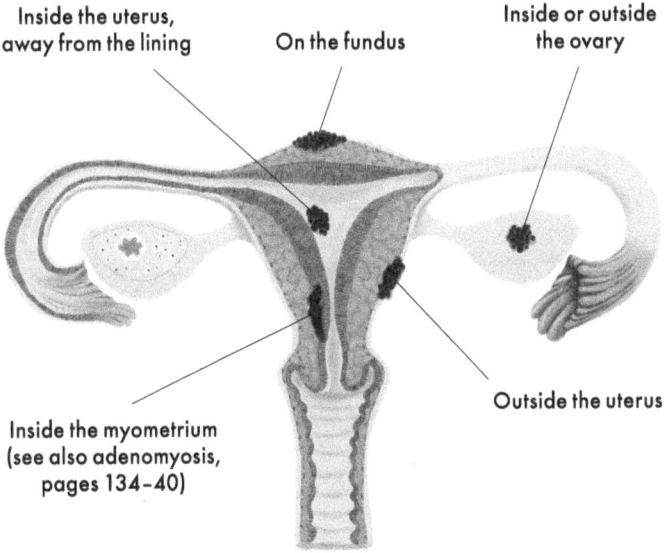

Inside the uterus,
away from the lining

On the fundus

Inside or outside
the ovary

Inside the myometrium
(see also adenomyosis,
pages 134–40)

Outside the uterus

Endometriosis in the bladder & bowel

Endometriosis is not exclusive to the reproductive system and the condition can cause cells similar to those in the endometrial lining to cluster on the bladder or bowel. In rare cases endometriosis can also spread as far as the heart and lungs (not pictured here). The diagram opposite shows some of the places where these cells can situate themselves.

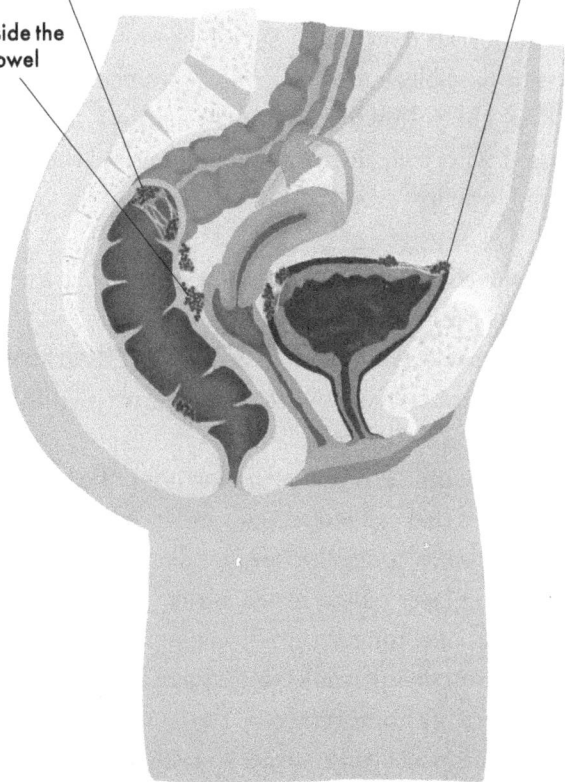

Inside the bowel

Outside the bladder

Outside the bowel

Treating endometriosis

Since there is no cure for endometriosis, treatment isn't straightforward. Some women opt for pain management to ease the symptoms and improve their quality of life, whereas others undergo surgery to prevent the condition from returning. Another way to prevent symptoms of endometriosis is to get pregnant which obviously may not always be possible or feasible for some women.

All of the following treatment options need to be discussed with your doctor, who will outline the various risks and benefits:

- **Pain relief** (paracetamol and/or ibuprofen, if the latter can be tolerated).
- **Hormone treatment** to slow the growth of the endometrial tissue (oral contraceptive pill, implant, injection or IUS coil).
- **Tranexamic acid**, a medication prescribed for heavy periods that can reduce pain and bleeding.
- **Ablation**, a surgical procedure that involves burning away a layer on the inside of the uterus, which can reduce or eliminate heavy bleeding.
- **Laparoscopic (keyhole) surgery** (see pages 78 and 150) for fertility improvement.
- **Precision excision surgery**, a surgical procedure in which a highly-skilled surgeon cuts away the adhesions.
- **Hysterectomy**, a surgical procedure to remove the womb and, in some cases, the cervix, the fallopian

tubes and the ovaries, to prevent the disease spreading further. A hysterectomy can provide symptom management but does not cure endometriosis.

My hope is that, in the future, with more research, endometriosis will be diagnosed easily and rapidly through the detection of bio markers – in other words, molecules found in blood, fluids or tissue that can flag up certain diseases or conditions. Endometriosis UK has a fabulous website for those needing more information (see Resources from page 203).

Living with endometriosis

The emotional and physical impact of endometriosis can be significant. The chronic pain can badly affect wellbeing, with work life, family life and social life often suffering as a consequence. Any difficulty you may have becoming pregnant – which may or may not be linked to the condition – will only pile on the pressure and trauma.

The lack of research means that, as things stand, we're unclear as to whether endometriosis directly causes infertility, although some do believe it may be associated with fertility problems, perhaps stemming from damage and scarring to reproductive organs. That being said, you shouldn't fear the worst if you receive an endometriosis diagnosis; even those with severe cases can go on to have a healthy baby.

Laparoscopic surgery for endometriosis

Laparoscopic (keyhole) surgery can be used to manage endometriosis. Under a general anaesthetic, a small incision is made into your abdomen and carbon dioxide gas is passed into the abdomen to inflate the area. The surgeon will then insert a laparoscope (a small telescope) through the incision in order to view the patches of endometriosis. These patches are then either surgically removed through a second incision or destroyed with electrosurgical heat treatment.

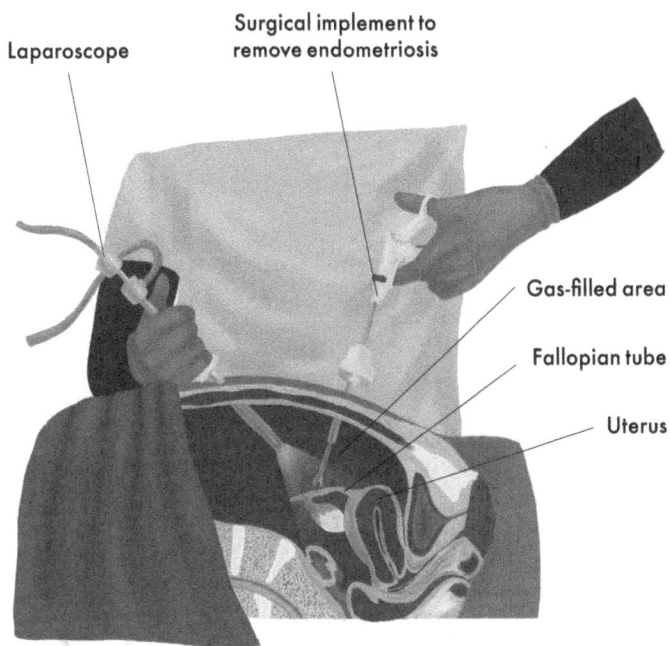

Laparoscope

Surgical implement to
remove endometriosis

Gas-filled area

Fallopian tube

Uterus

Uterine fibroids

Uterine fibroids (leiomyomas) are non-cancerous growths of the uterus. They're not associated with an increased risk of uterine cancer and do not usually develop into tumours. Fibroids vary hugely in size, from tiny growths that are invisible to the human eye, to really large masses that can be seen clearly on an ultrasound or MRI scan. A woman can develop a single fibroid or multiple fibroids; in extreme cases, a number of growths can expand into the uterus, adding weight to the abdomen and making you feel bloated, almost like you're pregnant.

Uterine fibroids are extremely common, so much so that one in three women will get them in their lifetime. We don't really know why they develop but we think it's linked to the hormone oestrogen, fluctuations of which can thicken the lining of the uterus, so they are more likely to occur during your fertile years when hormonal imbalances, variations or swings, especially of oestrogen, can be at their highest. Women who've had children have a lower risk of developing the condition, and the risk decreases with the more children you have. Fibroids tend to shrink as the menopause approaches and oestrogen levels decline. Those with Mediterranean or Afro-Caribbean heritage are said to be more susceptible to fibroids, as are obese or overweight women (excess weight causes an increased level of oestrogen in the body).

Symptoms of uterine fibroids

- Heavy periods.
- Painful periods.
- Stomach pain.
- Lower back pain.
- Bloating.
- Frequent need to urinate (as the mass presses on the bladder).
- Constipation.
- Pain or discomfort during sex.

Many people, however, don't even realize they have fibroids and often the growths will be shed with their uterine lining during menstruation.

In rarer cases, fibroids can hamper your chances of conceiving a baby, particularly if the fibroid is situated in the lining of the uterus and is somehow affecting implantation. The pregnancy itself can be affected by fibroids – they can hinder the growth of the baby – and, in some instances, they can cause infertility. Depending on their size and whereabouts, fibroids can act as 'foreign bodies', thus causing an obstruction between the egg and sperm or preventing implantation.

By age 35, 60% of Black women are thought to have uterine fibroids, compared to 6% of white women

Possible sites & types of uterine fibroids

Uterine fibroids are non-cancerous growths of the uterus and can vary hugely in size. There are several types of fibroid depending on their placement within the reproductive system: subserosal fibroids develop outside the wall of the uterus and grow into the pelvis; submucosal fibroids develop in the layer of muscle that lies beneath the lining of the uterus and can then push the walls of the uterus inwards; intramural fibroids develop inside the muscle walls of the uterus; intracavitary fibroids develop inside the cavity of the uterus; and pedunculated fibroids grow inside or outside the uterus, attached by a thin stalk of tissue.

GYNAECOLOGICAL AREAS OF CONCERN

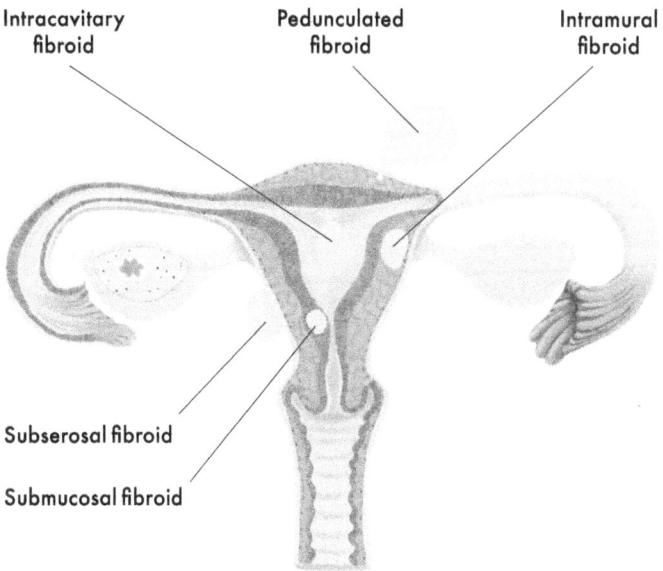

Intracavitary fibroid

Pedunculated fibroid

Intramural fibroid

Subserosal fibroid

Submucosal fibroid

Bi-manual examination for fibroids

Uterine fibroids are diagnosed with a bi-manual examination. During the examination the doctor will insert the fingers of one hand into the vaginal canal, place the other hand on the outside of the abdomen and palpate their hands in order to feel for fibroids inside or around the uterus.

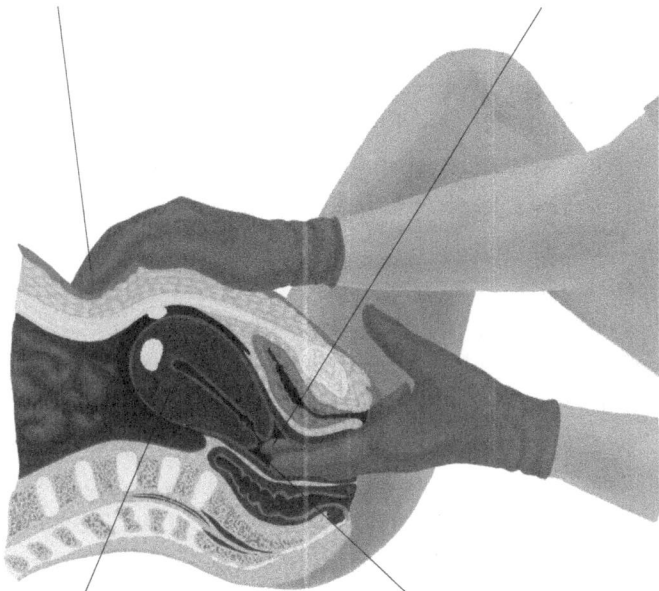

Pressing on the outside of the abdomen

Two fingers in the vagina, pressing upwards

Uterus

Vagina

Diagnosis of fibroids

If any of the symptoms listed on page 153 become problematic, speak to your doctor. They'll usually perform what's known as a bi-manual examination (see page 156), which involves palpating (feeling) the uterus to check for any bulkiness or any anomalies. Sometimes, patients will be referred for an ultrasound scan for further investigation.

Treatment of fibroids

Subsequent treatment depends on the site and severity of the fibroids. More often than not they don't need treating, since they shrink over time and are often shed with periods. Implementing lifestyle changes – like losing weight, stopping smoking and cutting down alcohol – can also help some women. The symptoms of pain and heavy bleeding can be managed by the combined oral contraceptive pill or the mini-pill (POP), or by LARCS (long-acting reversible contraceptives) such as the IUS progesterone coil, implant or injection. In more serious cases, we can try to shrink fibroids with hormone injections, or you can have minor surgery (fibroidectomy or myomectomy) to scrape away the lining of the uterus. The latter can be a suitable option if you're in your fertile years and are planning to have children.

A uterine ablation (a procedure to remove a thin layer of tissue) or a uterine fibroid embolization (when the blood supply to the fibroids is cut off) can also be performed, although the risks and benefits to your fertility would need to be weighed up by you and your clinician.

In extreme cases, a hysterectomy may be an option for those women who fully understand the implications of uterus-removal surgery.

Other issues

PCOS, adenomyosis, endometriosis and uterine fibroids are the more common (although still undiagnosed in many cases) conditions that can affect women in their fertile years, but there are a couple of more general conditions.

Pelvic inflammatory disease

Pelvic inflammatory disease (PID) is the general term for inflammation of the upper genital tract of the female reproductive system, including the uterus, the ovaries, the fallopian tubes and other connecting tissues. PID is often caused by a bacterial infection, which in many cases stems from a sexually transmitted disease (STD) such as chlamydia or gonorrhoea (see *The Power of Puberty & Periods*).

It's possible that PID can lead to pregnancy-related complications. Occasionally the fallopian tubes can be left narrowed and scarred, which may increase the chances of an ectopic pregnancy (see page 94). Someone with untreated or persistent PID may also be more likely to experience fertility issues; that being said, many of my patients who've had PID have been able to conceive and carry a baby without significant problems.

Early menopause

Early (or premature) menopause, which may occur for a variety of reasons, will have a significant impact on fertility and can affect your ability to have children naturally. There are more details about this in the third book of the series, *The Power of Menopause & Midlife.*

VULVAL & VAGINAL PAIN

Yvou may encounter pain in your vulva or vagina due to one of these conditions or as a result of FGM (see *The Power of Puberty & Periods*). Please also be aware that skin conditions in particular are often harder to diagnose among Black and Asian women with darker skin. Be persistent with your doctor if you are concerned!

Pelvic organ prolapse

Vaginal pain can occasionally be caused by a debilitating condition known as pelvic organ prolapse. This occurs when the uterus or the bladder slips down from its normal position and presses onto the vagina, causing a bulge.

A prolapse is not life-threatening but it can cause significant pain and discomfort, particularly in and around the vagina, making sex difficult and causing bladder leakage. While symptoms can vary in severity at different stages of your monthly cycle, or during or after exercise, sometimes they are ever-present.

Whereas pelvic organ prolapse is more likely to occur among post-menopausal women, it can also affect women in their twenties and thirties, particularly those with a high BMI (body mass index). Carrying extra weight can add pressure to the pelvic organs and can subsequently impact upon the vagina.

Symptoms of pelvic organ prolapse
- A feeling of heaviness around the lower abdomen and genitals.
- A visible lump or bulge in the vagina.
- Vaginal dryness.
- A dragging sensation in the vagina; some women say it feels like sitting on a small ball.
- Discomfort or numbness during sex.
- Difficulty passing urine.
- Urinary tract infection (UTI) symptoms such as burning when passing urine, pain on passing urine, blood in the urine, increased frequency of passing urine, incomplete emptying, passing more urine than usual at night, lower abdominal pain, fever.
- Abdominal discomfort.
- Backache.

Diagnosis of pelvic organ prolapse
If you're worried you have a prolapse, please get yourself checked out. Your doctor may perform an internal pelvic examination using a vaginal speculum or they'll do a bi-manual examination using both hands (see page 156). Sometimes your doctor will ask you to cough to see how pronounced the bulge is. They might also ask you to lie on your side in order to get a better view of the prolapse.

Treatment of pelvic organ prolapse

For milder cases, treatment is primarily related to implementing lifestyle changes and, as such, can take a while to have an effect.

- **Lose weight** if you're overweight, especially if your BMI is over 30. Your doctor will encourage you to follow a healthy eating plan.
- **Avoid heavy lifting** as much as possible, although I know this just isn't practical in real life – especially if you have children. Instead I ask my patients, as part of their rehab, to ask themselves, 'Do I need to be doing this lifting?' and to opt out if at all possible, perhaps delegating the task to someone else.
- **Follow a programme of specialized pelvic floor exercises** (see *The Power of Menopause & Midlife*), that your doctor can recommend. Pelvic floor muscle training helps to improve strength, endurance and coordination in that area (I often tell my patients to compare the pelvic floor with the foundations of a house – it provides stability and support for what is above). A programme of supervised physiotherapy is also suggested for at least 16 weeks for symptomatic women with grade 1 or 2 prolapses. Pilates can be very helpful, too, especially in the post-natal period.
- **Look after your bowel and bladder** by sitting on the toilet rather than hovering, so your muscles can relax. Try not to strain when you're having a poo; if you're

struggling to empty your bowels, perform a 'double voiding', which means having an initial wee, then standing up, then sitting back down before trying to poo again. To avoid constipation, preventative measures such as drinking more water and eating more fruit and vegetables may help, as well as taking laxatives if needed. You might even consider investing in a footstool so that you can position your body in a comfortable squatting position on the toilet, to aid healthy bowel movements. No need to rush things . . .just take your time!

- **Try topical vaginal oestrogen** to help with vaginal muscle tone, which can be affected by prolapses.

- **Use a vaginal pessary** if your pelvic organ prolapse is severe. A vaginal pessary is a soft, removable device (usually made from silicone) which is inserted inside the vagina in order to support the prolapsed walls of the vagina or uterus. It is usually inserted by a nurse or doctor, but some patients get the knack of inserting it themselves. Various shapes and sizes, such as ring pessaries or shelf pessaries, are available to suit individual needs. Women may choose a pessary for severe prolapses if they wish to avoid surgery but, on the downside, they can sometimes make sexual intercourse uncomfortable.

Some women don't respond well to preliminary treatment, and their quality of life suffers badly as a result. A doctor may decide to refer these patients to a gynaecologist,

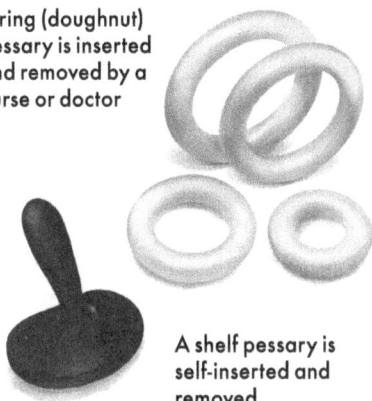

A ring (doughnut) pessary is inserted and removed by a nurse or doctor

A shelf pessary is self-inserted and removed

who will decide whether surgery is feasible. Options can include a sacrospinous fixation, which is an operation performed under general anaesthetic to stitch the top of the vagina or the cervix to a pelvic ligament, providing support to the pelvic floor. Vaginal mesh, which was once used to treat pelvic organ prolapse, is now banned in the UK. The other surgical option is a vaginal hysterectomy, a procedure that is less invasive than an abdominal hysterectomy and involves the removal of the cervix and the uterus via an incision in the vagina, thus removing the downward pressure of those organs. Your doctor should discuss the implications of uterus-removal surgery with you first.

Lichen sclerosus

Lichen sclerosus is a little-known, eczema-like skin condition that affects the vulva and perineum. It is not contagious.

Symptoms of lichen sclerosus

- Itchy red or white patches on the vulva or the perineum.
- Red, sore and inflamed, or bleeding (if rubbed) patches on the vulva or perineum.

Diagnosis of lichen sclerosus

Lichen sclerosus is usually diagnosed after examination by your doctor and discussion of your symptoms, although a biopsy may also be requested. If the patches change in size and shape, or are an enlarging lump that fails to heal, there is a small risk (around five per cent) of developing squamous cell carcinoma, a type of skin cancer. So it's imperative that you seek medical advice as soon as possible. I know no one relishes the idea of their genitalia being examined, but your health *must* outweigh any feelings of embarrassment. Your doctor will do all they can to make you feel as comfortable as possible and you can request a female doctor if you prefer.

Treatment of lichen sclerosus

- **Wearing cotton underwear** for better air flow.
- **Applying a vaginal moisturizer** and/or emollients.
- **Applying a prescribed steroid cream** (clobetasol propionate or diflucortolone valerate).
- **Using an oil-based vaginal lubricant** or a water-based vaginal moisturizer during sexual intercourse.
- **A prescribed low-dose neuropathic painkiller,** such as amitriptyline or gabapentin.

Effects of lichen sclerosus

Lichen sclerosus is a non-contagious, eczema-like skin condition on the vulva. It shows as itchy, sore white and/or red patches on the vulva or perineum and is more difficult to diagnose on darker skin. Below it is shown as white patches on the clitoral hood, clitoris, labia minora, perinium and rectum.

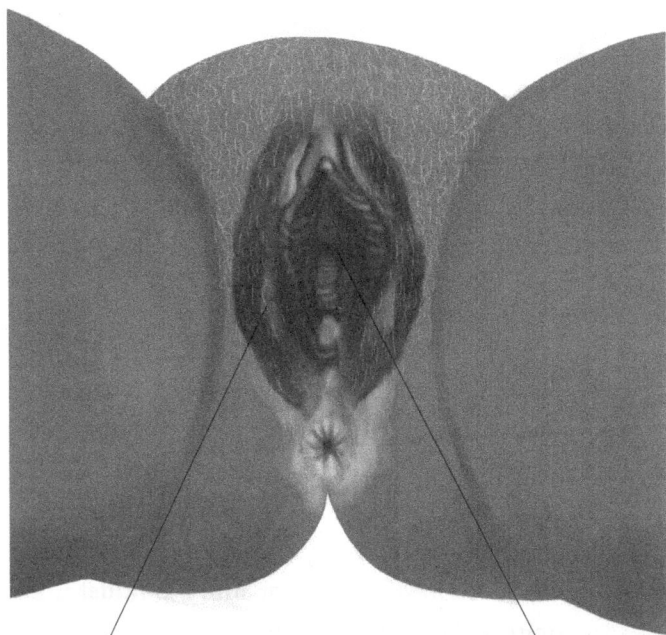

Itchy, white patches   Hardened, sore skin

Lichen planus

Lichen planus is a condition that can affect many areas of the skin including the vulva. It is not contagious and breastfeeding women can often suffer with lichen planus-like symptoms connected to hormone fluctuation.

Symptoms of lichen planus

- Soreness, burning and 'raw' sensation on the vulva.
- White streaks covering the vulva.
- Broken or split skin with painful red patches that can make sexual intercourse very uncomfortable.

Diagnosis of lichen planus

Lichen planus is usually diagnosed after examination by your doctor and discussion of your symptoms, although a biopsy may also be requested.

Treatment of lichen planus

- **Wearing cotton underwear** for better air flow.
- **Applying a vaginal moisturizer** and/or emollients.
- **Applying a prescribed steroid cream** (clobetasol propionate or diflucortolone valerate).
- **Using an oil-based vaginal lubricant** or a water-based vaginal moisturizer during sexual intercourse.
- **A prescribed low-dose neuropathic painkiller,** such as amitriptyline or gabapentin.
- **Low-dose vaginal oestrogen** (as a three-to-six-month course for breastfeeding women, or continual for perimenopausal women).

Effects of lichen planus

Lichen planus is a non-contagious skin condition on the vulva. Below it is shown as white streaks on the labia minora and sore patches around the vulva, clitoris and vagina.

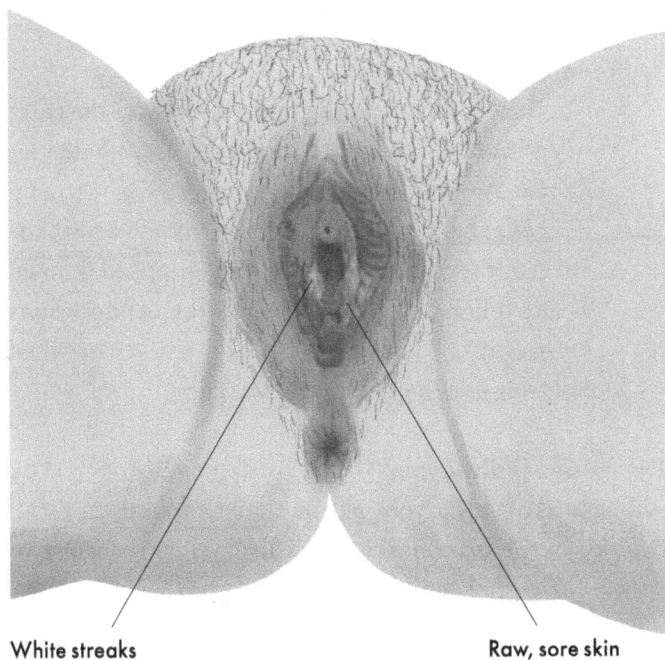

White streaks

Raw, sore skin

Vulvodynia

This condition is characterized by pain and discomfort in and around the vulval, vaginal and groin area, and can be classified as one of two types: unprovoked or generalized vulvodynia and provoked vulvodynia. Vulvodynia can be distressing, especially if you're in a sexual relationship, and it's believed that one-quarter of women will experience it at some point in their lives.

Symptoms of vulvodynia
- Continuous burning, stinging or soreness of the vulva or groin area (known as unprovoked vulvodynia, see lighter-coloured annotations on page 172).
- Pain experienced at the entrance to the vagina, the vulva or the clitoris when pressure is applied (known as provoked vulvodynia, see darker annotations on page 172). This may occur during sex or when inserting a tampon or menstrual cup.

Diagnosis of vulvodynia
A diagnosis of vulvodynia may be given by your doctor if all tests for infections come back negative, yet you continue to suffer with pain, burning or soreness.

Treatment of vulvodynia
There is no specific treatment for vulvodynia. Research into the condition is shockingly limited, but any underlying vulval/vaginal conditions such as vaginal atrophy (see *The Power of Menopause & Midlife*), lichen sclerosus

(see page 165) or lichen planus (see page 169) can be helped with a low dose of a medication called amitriptyline. The dose may be adjusted according to the response. The health and lifestyle tweaks for good vulval/vaginal health (see *The Power of Puberty & Periods*) should also help to alleviate symptoms.

Possible sites of vulvodynia

Unprovoked vulvodynia is a continuous soreness of the vulva (in the lighter-coloured areas below), while provoked vulvodynia (in the darker areas below) is pain felt when pressure is applied to the vulva, vagina, clitoris or groin.

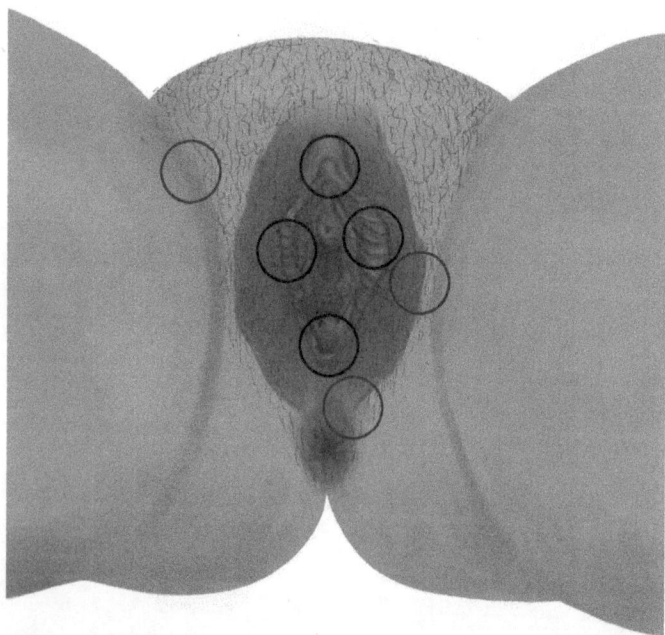

○ provoked vulvodynia

○ unprovoked vulvodynia

GYNAECOLOGICAL CANCERS

There are a number of gynaecological cancers that only affect women and trans people assigned female at birth and it is important to be aware of them. Being told you have cancer is everyone's worst nightmare. According to NHS research conducted in 2022, nearly six in ten of us admit that cancer is our greatest health fear, eclipsing other illnesses such as heart disease.

Prompt diagnosis is key to combatting this dreadful disease, of course, as is increased public awareness, and regular self examination is vital (see pages 31–35). However, far too many people with warning signs and tell-tale symptoms are reluctant to seek medical help by visiting their doctor. By putting things off – and perhaps convincing themselves they're okay, and that cancer only happens to other people – thousands of individuals each week are missing out on early, life-saving intervention.

In the survey, over two-fifths of people (42 per cent) admitted to putting off an appointment by either ignoring their symptoms, waiting to see if anything changed, looking for answers online or speaking to family and friends.

Your doctor wants to see you!
Please do not delay phoning for an appointment if you have a persistent problem that's been playing on your mind. You may be losing weight for no apparent reason,

for example, or you may be aware of a lump in your breast or a sore on your vulva. It might be nothing serious, but you're not losing anything by getting checked out by a clinician.

If something doesn't feel right to you and doesn't seem better after three weeks, please see your doctor. Keep a diary if you can to track your symptoms: keep track of your period, your eating habits, your weight, your bowel movements. And when you speak to the receptionist, have the confidence to say 'I'm bleeding between periods and I'm scared it might be cervical cancer', because your specific concerns will then be flagged up to the doctor. Being forewarned in this way will help your doctor to zone in on your symptoms and optimize that initial appointment.

As a doctor with a specialist interest in women's health, I'm particularly keen to raise awareness of the five main gynaecological cancers:

- Ovarian
- Vulval
- Vaginal
- Cervical
- Uterine

It can be very difficult to spot the warning signs associated with these cancers, especially ovarian cancer. Because of this, some women can receive a relatively late diagnosis – at stage 3 or stage 4, when the disease is severe with a poor prognosis. Tragically, many will lose their lives. Gynaecological cancer mortality rates need to be reduced, and doctors like myself are doing our utmost to encourage women to recognize the key symptoms and seek the appropriate help.

Where gynaecological cancers can occur

There are five main gynaecological cancers. These areas are highlighted opposite and it is possible for cancerous cells to grow in the uterus (uterine cancer), one or both ovaries (ovarian cancer), the cervix (cervical cancer), the vagina (vaginal cancer) or the vulva (vulval cancer).

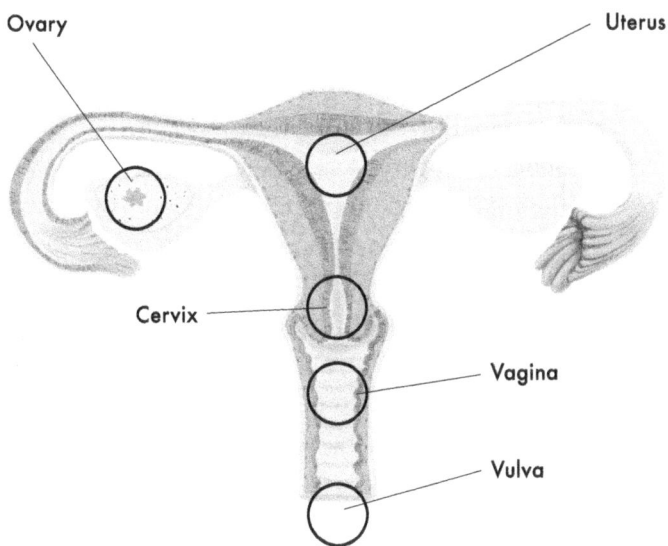

Ovary

Uterus

Cervix

Vagina

Vulva

Potential gynaecological concerns: what symptoms might warrant a visit to your doctor?

The main symptoms to watch out for are as follows (and just one of these may be a sign of cancer):

- **Abnormal vaginal bleeding** (which is unrelated to your menstrual cycle).
- **Abnormal vaginal discharge** (unlike your usual clear, white odourless secretion).
- **Changes in appetite** – such as feeling full too quickly or loss of appetite – that continue for more than three weeks.
- **Weight loss** that is unexplained by lifestyle changes.
- **Itching, burning, tenderness or sensitivity** in the vulva or vagina.
- **Changes of skin colour** in the vulva.
- **Rashes, lesions, sores or warts** in the vulva.
- **New moles (or changes to existing moles)** in the vulva or vagina.
- **Lumps or bumps** in the vulva or vagina.
- **Pelvic pain** or pressure.
- **Pain and/or bleeding** during or after sexual intercourse.
- **More frequent urgency to urinate** and/or painful urination.
- **Constipation.**
- **Persistent bloating** (for longer than three weeks).

- Abdominal pain.
- Back pain.

There are some great tools and resources offering gynaecological cancer support online (see Resources from page 203).

Cervical screening (smear tests)

Millions of women around the world die of cervical cancer each year, so it's really important that you minimize your risk by attending your regular cervical screening appointment. Commonly known as a smear, this test checks for HPV (human papillomavirus) as well as early cervical cell changes and is offered every three years to women aged between 25 and 49, and every five years for those aged between 50 and 65. If you have already had the HPV vaccine (see *The Power of Puberty & Periods*) you must still attend, as must those who've never had sexual intercourse. This is really important as it is still commonly (and incorrectly) believed that cervical screening is only relevant if you have had sexual contact, and we know that in some cultures pre-marital sex or loss of virginity has a lot of stigma attached to it, which can in turn lead women to avoid having a smear test. If you are a trans or non-binary person with a cervix, and are aged between 25 and 65, you should have a smear test. If you're registered as male with your healthcare provider you may not receive an automatic invite, so check with your surgery that you're listed on their call and recall system.

The smear test takes just a few minutes to perform – either by a nurse or doctor – and patients usually receive their results around two to six weeks later. You may ask for the test to be performed by a clinician of a certain gender (although this isn't always possible) and request a chaperone.

Preparing for a smear test
It's normal to feel anxious about your cervical screening, especially if it's your first time as the 'fear of the unknown' can be concerning. Please don't let this prevent you from attending this potentially life-saving procedure. Speaking with your nurse or doctor beforehand can be really helpful, since measures can be taken to make smear tests more comfortable. Here are some key points:

- Try to book your smear test at a time when you're not on your period; towards the middle or end of your cycle is ideal.
- Several weeks before your appointment, it's a good idea to start using a topical, water-based vaginal moisturizer to maximize lubrication. You may even want to take some along to the screening.
- Midlife or older women who suffer with vaginal dryness as a result of vaginal atrophy (see *The Power of Menopause & Midlife*), vulvo-vaginal pain or lichen sclerosus (see page 165) may also use topical localized vaginal oestrogen HRT at least one month before their appointment. This medication improves the general health and flexibility of the vaginal walls, which can make the smear test more comfortable. It does not cause or increase the risk of breast cancer,

as it gets absorbed directly into the local area as opposed to the bloodstream (it can even be used by women who have, or have had, breast cancer). You can ask your doctor or nurse to prescribe vaginal oestrogen for you in advance.

- You must stop using vaginal oestrogen HRT, oil-based lubricants or spermicides two days before.
- If you have any other physical or psychological concerns – you may have had an episiotomy, for example, or survived FGM or sexual trauma – then please speak to your doctor or nurse beforehand.
- Any patients with mobility issues – you may be a wheelchair user, or have severe back pain – may also want to discuss their options in advance.
- If you prefer, you may request a chaperone to accompany you during a smear test; please speak to your surgery beforehand if this is the case.

What happens at a smear test

As someone who's performed countless smear tests, I can reassure you that it's a safe and simple procedure that should only take a couple of minutes. Here's a run-down of what to expect:

- First of all, you'll be given some privacy and asked to remove your underwear.
- You'll then be asked to lie on a bed with your knees bent, and with your legs open. There may be stirrups into which you can place your heels.

- Once you're comfortable, the nurse or doctor will carefully insert a plastic or metal speculum into your vagina. For ease of passage, they should use a water-based lubricant, which might feel cold at first.
- The speculum is gently inserted sideways, then rotated. Then it is opened up to allow vision and access to the cervix (neck of the uterus). The speculum might make a sound when it is adjusted.
- A long, slender plastic device called a cervix brush, or a swab, is inserted and used to carefully collect the cells on the outer wall of the cervix.
- The brush and speculum are gently removed from the vagina, and you are able to close your legs.
- You'll then be given some privacy to wipe yourself with paper provided, before getting dressed.
- The clinician will place the brush into a sample pot, which will be sent to a laboratory for investigation.

Your comfort should be paramount during a screening – clinicians should do their utmost to make you feel relaxed – but if at any point during your smear test you have any concerns, or do not wish to continue, please make this clear to your healthcare professional. For example, do not be afraid to ask the nurse or doctor, 'Are you using a lubricant on the speculum?' and, if they're not – or don't have any – you have the right to refuse to proceed with the test. You can then ask the surgery to rebook another smear test as soon as possible or to be referred to a specialist clinic (please don't just abandon things, though; you *must* keep that appointment).

Once the test is complete the sample will be sent for testing and you will be told when to expect the results. If no HPV cells are found then no further testing is needed and you should attend your next smear test in three or five years' time. If HPV cells are detected you will either be asked to go for another smear test in a year's time for the doctor to monitor the HPV cells, or you may be referred for a colposcopy, which is a similar process to a smear test and performed in a hospital.

Preventative care: look after yourself

Cancer is a cruel, indiscriminate disease that can affect people of all ages and backgrounds. It's the cause of one in four deaths in the UK alone, and one in two of us will be affected by it in our lifetimes. In some cases, cancer can be difficult to prevent if you possess an inherited gene. However, in other cases, preventative measures can really help to lessen your chance of getting the disease. I'd be *so* happy if you and your loved ones could consider the following lifestyle changes. They may go a long way towards minimizing your risk, and may help fend off other illnesses, too.

- **Keep your weight down** (preferably BMI below 25).
- **Take regular exercise** (it doesn't have to be strenuous or expensive . . . 120 minutes per week of walking, cycling or yoga is great).

- **Stop smoking** (see page 64).
- **Cut down or cut out alcohol** (women should consume no more than 14 units per week).
- **Minimize stress** (look at ways to reduce anxiety, like listening to music, mindfulness or meditation).

Having a smear test

The smear test is the routine screening to check the cervix and try to prevent cervical cancer by detecting HPV cells. For the test you will undress from the waist down and the doctor or nurse will insert a speculum (a smooth device) into your vagina. Once in place the speculum is gently widened to allow the doctor or nurse to view the cervix. They then gently wipe a small brush, or swab, over the cervix to collect a sample of cells. Once the sample is collected the speculum will be unwound and removed and you'll be given an opportunity to get dressed in privacy.

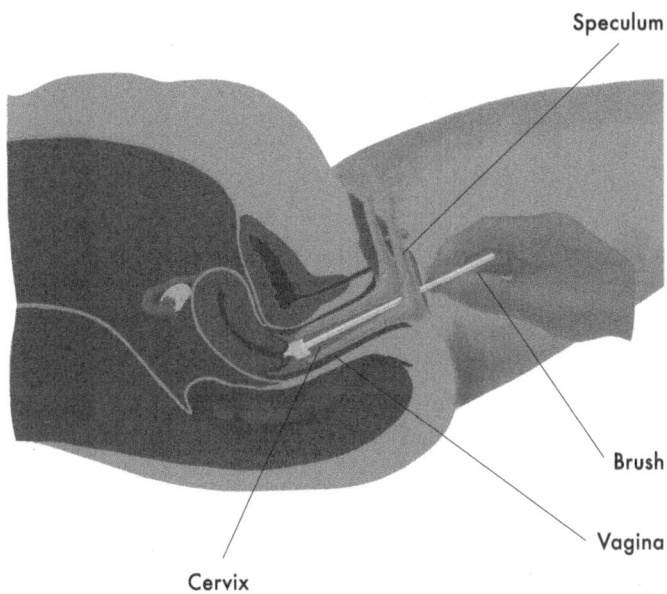

Speculum

Brush

Vagina

Cervix

DR NIGHAT'S TAKEAWAYS

1 Be mindful that things don't always go to plan
If you are planning a pregnancy, give yourself the best chance of conceiving by having unprotected vaginal sex every two to three days.

2 If you have had difficulty conceiving for one year . . .
book a double appointment with your doctor (with your partner if possible) to discuss further investigations.

3 Register with the community midwife
As soon as you know you are pregnant, register with the midwife to get your booking appointment. Take folic acid and vitamin D throughout your pregnancy and until you finish breastfeeding.

4 Don't miss those screenings
Ensure that you're registered with your healthcare provider for screenings. Make a note of the frequency and call for an appointment if you think you're past due. It's vitally important that you attend, so don't miss out!

5 Keep practising self-care!
Examining your own body is crucial in the fight against breast, vulval and vaginal cancer (see pages 19–35 for a full breakdown of self-examinations). So check your pair, then check down there!

SHARING THE KNOWLEDGE

Throughout our lives we need to be able to keep checking and understanding our bodies. Know what is normal for you. Understand when something is not right and know when to go to your doctor to show your concern.

I want to emphasize that the stigma and taboo around women's health and women's biology ends with this book. Enough with the lack of diversity and inclusion in medical textbooks. Enough with misrepresentation of neurodiverse women and those who are differently abled. Enough of ignoring ethnic minority communities. Enough of undermining and gaslighting women's bodies and their symptoms. Enough with not providing adequate pain relief for smear tests, childbirth and hysteroscopies. Enough of not showing real-life body shapes. Enough of lack of data. Enough of medical misogyny, which is perpetrated by the patriarchy – including the patriarchy within us and our own misgivings about whether our pain is worth discussing.

Hopefully by now you've recognized that I have absolutely no qualms talking about breasts, vulvas, vaginas, anuses – the lot! I think it's so important for women to be queens of their bodies, and as queens we should be fixing each other's crowns along the way.

This book is not mine; it is my gift to you. Take the

knowledge within this book and share it like confetti with those around you.

Dr Nighat Arif

This book is my gift to you: take it, look after it, come back to it when you're ready, and know that you have the freedom to choose the care that suits you.

GLOSSARY OF WOMEN'S HEALTH

Abdomen The region of the body between the chest and the pelvis that contains the digestive and reproductive (or abdominal) organs, often referred to as the belly.

Abortion The termination of a pregnancy before term; this can be medically induced or spontaneous (known as miscarriage).

Adenoma A non-cancerous cyst or tumour resembling glandular tissue arising from the layer of cells inside organs (epithelium).

Adenomyosis A condition in which the cells that normally line the uterine walls (endometrium) develop in the muscular wall of the uterus tissue, but continue to thicken and shed as part of the menstrual cycle. Unlike endometriosis, these cells are always inside the uterus.

Amniotic fluid The clear, watery fluid that surrounds a foetus in the uterus, cushioning it as the mother moves around and allowing the foetus to move freely.

Amniotic sac The membranous 'bag' surrounding a foetus in the uterus, which is filled with amniotic fluid.

Anaemia A condition in which the concentration of the oxygen-carrying pigment (haemoglobin) in red blood cells is too low. It can result because there are insufficient red blood cells or because those that are circulating are defective. It is not a disease, but a feature of different disorders.

Anaesthetic Literally means loss of sensation. In medicine, anaesthetics are used to numb sensation in certain areas (local anaesthetic), or to induce sleep, for example for surgery (general anaesthetic).

Anal sex A form of sex in which a man's penis enters the anal passage of his partner.

Androgen Hormone that promotes the development and maintenance of male characteristics.

Antenatal Literally the time before birth of a baby. The term is mostly used to describe the care a mother receives during pregnancy prior to the birth.

Antibiotic drugs A group of drugs used to treat bacterial infections. They are sometimes offered to prevent infection if the immune system is impaired.

Bacteria (single = bacterium) Single-celled organisms abundant in air, soil and water, that are mostly harmless to humans. Some, such as gut bacteria, are beneficial and help break down food. A few, so-called pathogens, can cause disease.

Barrier method of contraception Forms of birth control, such as a condom or cap, that physically prevent a sperm reaching an egg.

Benign A growth or tumour that is not cancerous. It may continue to grow in situ, but it will not spread to other parts of the body.

Bilateral salpingo-oophorectomy Surgical procedure in which the ovaries and fallopian tubes are removed, often carried out as keyhole surgery.

Bi-manual examination A form of examination used to check internal organs in which the practitioner places one hand on the lower part of the person's abdomen and at the same time inserts two fingers into their vagina.

Biopsy A diagnostic test in which a small amount of tissue or a few cells are removed from the body for microscopic examination.

Birth control Any means of controlling fertility to prevent pregnancy, commonly described as contraception.

Bloating A feeling of fullness or swelling in the abdomen, possibly as a result of gas in the intestines, overeating, food intolerances or constipation.

Blood clot A mass of blood that forms if blood platelets, proteins and cells stick together. It can be carried around the body in the bloodstream or can become attached to the wall of a blood vessel (thrombus).

Body mass index (BMI) A means of assessing whether a person is a healthy weight by measuring both weight and height – weight in kg/lbs is divided by height in metres/inches squared – then plotting the calculation on a chart, which gives a number, for example anything between 18.5–24.9 is a healthy weight, above 25 is overweight and above 30 is obese.

Caesarean section/delivery Also called a C-section, this is an operation to deliver a baby through an incision in the abdomen. It is usually performed if a vaginal delivery is medically risky or because a birth becomes difficult (emergency Caesarean).

Cardiovascular disease Disorders and diseases that affect the heart and blood vessels.

Cervical mucus The slippery discharge secreted by the cervix that makes it easier for sperm to swim up the vagina; its consistency changes during the menstrual cycle.

Cervical screening A regular screening test offered every 3–5 years in women aged 25–65 that assesses the health of the cervix. Cells are taken from the cervix to check for types of human papillomavirus (HPV) that can cause cancerous changes.

Cervix The opening in the lower end of the uterus that leads to the vagina.

Chaperone A person who accompanies another, for example to a medical appointment.

Cisgender (cis) A person whose gender identity is the same as that identified at birth.

Clitoris Part of the female genitalia, this is a small sensitive erectile organ located just below the pubic bone, partly enclosed by the labia.

Clot *see* blood clot

Coeliac disease A condition in which the small intestine is hypersensitive to gluten, the protein found in wheat, rye and barley. Eating gluten causes the immune system to attack and damage the gut tissues, and as a result the person cannot absorb nutrients.

Cognitive function Term used to describe mental processes involved with the acquisition of knowledge, information processing and reasoning.

Coil A small T-shaped device inserted in the uterus to prevent pregnancy. There are two types: a copper coil (intra-uterine device or IUD) and a hormone-releasing coil (intra-uterine system or IUS).

Combined oral contraceptive pill Contraception in the form of a pill that contains artificial versions of the naturally occurring hormones progesterone and oestrogen.

Conception The beginning of pregnancy marked by the fertilization of an egg (ovum) by a sperm.

Condom A sheath-shaped barrier device used to prevent pregnancy and prevent sexually transmitted infections. Condoms can be placed over the penis, or female versions (femidoms) are inserted into the vagina.

Contraception A means of controlling fertility to prevent pregnancy with barrier methods, coils or hormones.

Contraceptive injection An injection that releases the hormone progesterone into the bloodstream for longer-term pregnancy prevention; the effects can last between 8 and 13 weeks depending on the type.

Contraceptive implant Long-term form of contraception in which a small, flexible plastic rod is placed under the skin.

Contractions, uterine Rhythmic spasms of the muscles in the walls of the uterus that occur during childbirth.

Copper coil A small T-shaped implement inserted into the uterus as a form of contraception. This can be fitted at any point in the menstrual cycle.

Corpus luteum A cyst, or cluster of cells, which develops in the ovary during every menstrual cycle, just after an egg (ovum) leaves the ovary.

Crabs *see* Pubic lice

Cramps, period Known as dysmenorrhoea, cramps are painful sensations that can occur when the body releases the hormone-like substances called prostaglandins that cause the uterus to contract to expel its lining before and during a menstrual period.

Cyclical HRT A form of hormone replacement therapy (HRT) offered to women who have menopausal symptoms but who also still have their periods.

Depression A mood disorder that results in persistent feelings of sadness and hopelessness. Symptoms vary depending on the severity.

Diabetes A long-term metabolic disease characterized by high levels of blood sugar (glucose) in the body. Blood sugar is usually broken down by the hormone insulin. Diabetes can develop because the body produces no insulin (Type 1) or because the body cannot use the insulin it produces (Type 2) – the latter is often reversible.

Gestational diabetes A form of diabetes that can develop in pregnancy; this often resolves after pregnancy.

Diagnosis The process of identifying the nature of an illness by examination and assessment of the symptoms.

Diaphragm A barrier method of contraception that is fitted into the vagina to cover the cervix before vaginal sex.

Discharge Fluid that comes out of the body.

Early menopause This is the onset of menopause before the age of 40, and is also known as premature menopause or premature ovarian insufficiency (POI).

Egg A mature female reproductive cell (ovum) released from an ovary that, if fertilized, can develop into an embryo.

Ejaculation The action of ejecting semen from a male's body.

Embryo Human offspring in the process of development from fertilized egg to a foetus.

Emergency contraception This is contraception that can be given after unprotected sex to prevent a pregnancy. There are two forms: a person can take the morning-after pill, or a coil can be inserted.

Endometriosis A condition that occurs when microscopic cells similar to those found in the lining of the uterus – known as the endometrium – are distributed outside the uterus.

Endometrium The inner lining of the uterus.

Episiotomy A surgical cut that can be made at the entrance of the vagina to help a difficult birth and prevent perineum tearing.

Fallopian tube One of two tubes that extend from the top of the uterus towards the ovaries, in which fertilization takes place. The ovum moves along the tube towards the main body of the uterus and the sperm travels from the uterus towards the tube.

Family planning, *see* Contraception

Fasting cholesterol test A blood test to check for cholesterol levels, for which the person is normally asked not to eat for 12 hours beforehand.

Fertility A person or couple's ability to produce offspring, which is dependent on age and health.

Fertilization The point at which a sperm enters an egg (ovum).

Fibroid A benign, slow-growing tumour formed of smooth muscle and connective tissue that can develop in the uterus. There can be one or more and the size can vary.

Follicle A small cavity in the body, for example a hair follicle. In an ovary, follicles are small sac-like, fluid-filled pouches, each of which contains one ovum (egg).

GP A general practitioner, or family doctor, is a doctor who assesses and treats common medical conditions, and refers patients to other medical disciplines for more specialist treatment when necessary.

Gender The sex that a person identifies themselves as, such as male, female or non-binary.

Gender affirmation therapy Any of several therapies, psychological and physical, that are offered to a person to help them live in their preferred gender identity.

Gender diverse A place that accommodates people of different genders; also an umbrella term used to address the spectrum of different gender identities.

Genitals A person's external sex organs.

Gestation The period of time between conception and birth during which an infant develops in the uterus, normally 40 weeks or 9 months.

Gynaecological cancer A cancer that affects any part of the reproductive system of a female.

Gynaecologist Doctor or surgeon specializing in the branch of medicine that focuses on female health and the female reproductive system.

Hormone Chemical messengers released into the bloodstream by certain organs that have a specific effect on tissues somewhere else in the body.

Hot flush A common symptom of the menopause, caused by hormonal imbalances, in which a person experiences a sudden rise in body temperature especially in the upper body, often accompanied by sweating, and looks flushed.

Hyperthyroidism Also known as overactive thyroid, a condition that results in overproduction of thyroid hormones. Symptoms include increase in heart rate, appetite and sweating, as well as weight loss.

Hypothyroidism Also known as underactive thyroid, a condition that results in inadequate levels of thyroid hormones, causing tiredness, lethargy and weight gain.

Hysterectomy The surgical removal of the uterus. The most common type involves only the uterus and cervix; sometimes the ovaries and fallopian tubes are also removed.

Implantation The point at which a fertilized egg (ovum) attaches itself to the wall of the uterus – this normally happens six days after fertilization.

Incontinence The involuntary passing of urine, which can be caused by injury, weakness or disease of the urinary tract.

Infertility Inability to produce a baby. This can be a result of a problem in the male or female reproductive systems, or both.

Inflammation Pain, swelling, heat and redness in one or several areas of the body as a result of an injury or infection.

Insomnia The inability to fall asleep or to stay asleep for any length of time. Causes can be physical, psychological or environmental.

Insulin The hormone produced by the pancreas that controls blood sugar levels in the body.

Insulin resistance A condition in which the body's cells do not respond properly to insulin whether it's produced by the body, or injected (in those with diabetes).

Intercourse Also known as sexual intercourse, this is physical contact between two individuals that involves genitalia of at least one of them.

Intra-uterine device (IUD) Small 'T'-shaped, non-hormonal device (coil) that is inserted into the uterus as a form of contraception.

Intra-uterine system (IUS) Small 'T'-shaped, hormone-releasing device (coil) that is inserted into the uterus as a form of contraception.

Keloid scars A scar that continues growing after a wound is healed and can grow to bigger than the original wound.

LGBTQ+ Acronym used to refer to the group of people who identify as lesbian, gay, bisexual, transgender, queer or questioning. The '+' acknowledges that there are other sexual identities, such as intersex and asexual.

Labia majora The outer lips of the female external genitals.

Labia minora The inner lips of the female external genitals.

Labour The process by which an infant is born.

Laparoscopy A surgical procedure in which the interior of the abdomen is examined using a device called a laparoscope, which is inserted through a small hole ('key' hole) made in the abdominal wall.

Libido Level of sexual desire.

Lubricant An oily or slippery substance that can for example be used to reduce friction during intercourse.

MRI scan Short for magnetic resonance imaging, this is a diagnostic technique that produces cross-sectional or three-dimensional images of organs or body structures.

Mammogram A type of X-ray used specifically to examine the breasts for signs of cancer, offered as a form of screening.

Mastectomy Surgical removal of one or both breasts, usually to treat breast cancer.

Menopause The point in a woman's life when menstruation has ceased for 12 months, regardless of other symptoms.

Menstruation The periodic shedding of the lining of a woman's uterus that occurs if they are not pregnant.

Midwife A person trained to assist women in childbirth.

Migraine A type of headache characterized by recurrent attacks of severe pain, usually on one side of the head, which can cause a throbbing sensation.

Mini-pill Also known as the progesterone-only pill (POP), this is a contraceptive pill that contains only progesterone, which works by thickening the cervical mucus and preventing the sperm reaching the egg.

Miscarriage The loss of a foetus before week 24 of pregnancy.

Morning-after pill, *see* Emergency contraception

Multidisciplinary team Healthcare team that is comprised of a number of different specialties, who work together to assist with a person's medical care.

Myometrium The muscle tissue in the wall of the uterus.

Nausea Feeling sick or the need to vomit.

Needlestick injury Accidental puncture of the skin by a potentially contaminated hypodermic needle, which carries a risk of disease.

Neuropathic or neuropathy Disease or inflammation affecting the peripheral nerves, the nerves that connect to the central nervous system (brain and spinal cord).

NHS The UK's health system – the National Health Service – which includes all healthcare practitioners.

Non-binary A person who does not identify themselves as either male or female.

Obesity A state of being very overweight; a person with a BMI above 30 is described as obese.

Obstetrician A doctor or surgeon specializing in the branch of medicine concerned with childbirth.

Oestrogen(s) A group of hormones essential for the maintenance of female characteristics of the body.

Oestrogen-receptor-positive breast cancer (ER+) A type of breast cancer with cells that have receptors that allow them to use oestrogen hormones to grow – so a person can be given medication to reduce the hormone production as a form of treatment.

Off licence Use of a drug or other preparation in a way that is not typically recommended by the manufacturer, but that is still safe.

Oophorectomy Surgical procedure in which the ovaries are removed.

Oral medication Medicines or tablets that are taken by mouth.

Oral sex Sexual activity in which one person's genitals are stimulated by the mouth of another person.

Osteoporosis Loss of bone tissue that causes bones to become brittle/fragile so are more likely to fracture. This is a natural part of ageing, but women lose bone tissue faster after the menopause.

Ovarian cyst Abnormal, fluid-filled swelling that can develop on an ovary.

Ovary One of two glands, positioned either side of the uterus, in which eggs (ova) form and the female hormones oestrogen and progesterone are made.

Ovulation The process of the ovary releasing an egg (ovum).

Ovum (plural = ova) The mature female reproductive cell released from an ovary that, if fertilized, can develop into an embryo.

Patch An adhesive-plaster-like device that releases medication, for example for HRT or contraception, into the body through the skin; the patch is normally changed every 2–3 weeks.

Pelvis Large bony, basin-like frame at the base of the spine that surrounds and protects the reproductive organs.

Penetration Physical contact between two individuals in which a man puts his penis into the vagina or anus of their partner.

Penis The largest external male sex organ.

Perimenopause The time before the menopause when a woman has symptoms of the menopause, but is still menstruating; this can last up to a decade.

Perinatal phase The weeks immediately before and after the birth of a baby.

Perineum The part of the body between the entrance to the vagina (or the scrotum) and the anus.

Period Also known as menstruation, this is the periodic shedding of the lining of a woman's uterus that occurs if they are not pregnant.

Pessary Medical device placed into the vagina, to correct the position of the uterus or to deliver medication or contraception.

Physiotherapist Healthcare professional who provides physical therapy treatment to help prevent or reduce joint stiffness and aid movement.

Pituitary gland Situated under the brain, this is the most important gland of the endocrine (hormone-producing) system. Called the master gland, it controls and regulates all the other endocrine glands and many body processes.

Placenta The organ formed in the uterus during pregnancy that supports and nourishes the foetus.

Placental abruption Separation of the placenta from the wall of the uterus during pregnancy or labour before the baby is born; this is life-threatening to mother and baby.

Polyp A growth, often from a stalk, that projects from the wall of an organ, such as the cervix, uterus, or nose. Some are cancerous and need to be removed.

Polycystic ovary syndrome (PCOS) A condition that can cause cysts on the ovaries. Confusingly the syndrome can also cause other effects (such as excess hair, weight gain, oily skin, or irregular or absent periods) without the presence of cysts on the ovaries.

Post-menopause The life stage of a woman, or person assigned a woman at birth, after the menopause.

Post-natal The first weeks after the birth of a baby.

Post-partum The hours immediately after the birth of a baby.

Premature menopause Menopause that begins when a woman is under the age of 40 years.

Progesterone Hormone made in the ovaries that is essential to the functioning of the female reproductive system.

Progesterone-only pill (POP) *see* Mini pill

Progestogen drugs A group of drugs containing properties similar to naturally occurring hormone progesterone that are used in contraceptives.

Prolapse Displacement of an organ, for example the uterus, from its normal place in the body.

Puberty The time during which a girl (or boy) becomes sexually mature.

Pubic lice Tiny parasitic insects, often called crabs, that can attach themselves to the skin and hair of the areas around the genitals. Spread by close physical contact they cause intense itching; lice and/or eggs may be visible.

Pulmonary embolism Obstruction of one of the arterial blood vessels in the lungs by a blood clot. Clots can form in the lungs or be carried there from another part of the circulatory system by the blood.

Screening The regular testing of apparently healthy members of the population to check for signs of diseases.

Semen The sperm-containing fluid released from the penis during ejaculation/ orgasm.

Sequential HRT A form of hormone replacement therapy for women who still menstruate that involves taking one hormone daily (oestrogen), then additional progesterone for part (normally half) of the month.

Sexuality A person's identity in relation to the genders they are attracted to, and/or how they identify their own sexuality. It also describes a person's attitude and behaviour towards sex and physical intimacy with others.

Sexually transmitted diseases (STDs) Diseases that are transmitted through sexual contact with another person.

Side effect The secondary response caused by a drug beyond the intended therapeutic effects.

Smear test Routine screening test offered every 3–5 years to all women (or those assigned female at birth) aged 25–65 in which cells are collected from the cervix to check for types of human papillomavirus (HPV) that can cause cancerous changes in the cervix.

Speculum Device placed in the vagina by a healthcare professional so that the cervix can be checked, and a smear test can be carried out.

Sperm The male sex cell that is responsible for fertilization of an egg (ovum).

Spotting Light traces of blood that can indicate the end of a period, or that are sometimes seen around ovulation.

Stress incontinence Involuntary loss of urine that occurs, for example, when a person coughs or lifts a heavy object, because the muscles at the exit to the urinary tract (sphincter) are weakened, for example after childbirth.

Surrogacy The process of carrying and giving birth to a baby for another person. The birth mother then hands over custody of the baby to that person.

Swab Small absorbent pad or cloth (generally sterile) used in surgery or by a healthcare professional to clean a wound, apply medication or take a specimen.

Synthetic A chemically made substance that imitates a naturally occurring product.

Systemic Medical treatment using substances/drugs that travel throughout the body.

Testosterone The hormone that stimulates the development of, and maintains, secondary male characteristics.

Tinnitus Continuous or intermittent ringing, buzzing or roaring sound in one, or more commonly both, ears.

Topical A medication or treatment applied directly to an area (of skin, for example).

Toxic shock syndrome A rare, but potentially life-threatening, condition caused by harmful bacteria getting into the body and releasing toxins. It is sometimes associated with tampon use in young women.

Trans man Person living as a man who was assigned female gender at birth.

Trans woman Person living as a woman who was assigned male gender at birth.

Transdermal Application of a drug through the skin, typically via an adhesive patch.

Transgender, or trans A person who is not living as the gender they were assigned at birth.

Transvaginal ultrasound scan An ultrasound scan carried out using a probe inserted into the vagina, *see also* Ultrasound scan

Trimester One of the three 'periods' of pregnancy, each covering around one-third of the pregnancy.

Triple-negative cancer An aggressive, fast-growing form of breast cancer in which the cells do not have hormone receptors that they need for growth.

Ultrasound scan A diagnostic tool that involves passing high-frequency sound waves through the body – the reflected echoes build a picture of the organs, or foetus for example, visible on a screen.

Unprotected sex Sexual intercourse with no form of contraception.

Urethra The opening, or sphincter, at the end of the ureter through which urine flows out of the body.

Urge incontinence The uncontrolled leakage of urine that occurs when a person feels a sudden urge to pee and is unable to stop the flow.

Uterine fibroids (leiomyomas) Noncancerous growths of the uterus.

Uterus Largest internal female reproductive organ in which a foetus remains during pregnancy.

Vaccine A medical preparation that is given to induce immunity to an infectious disease. Some require several doses to take effect and for others one dose provides life immunity.

Vagina The muscular tube, or canal, between the external female genitalia (vulva) and the internal organs of the cervix and the uterus.

Vaginal mucus Slimy substance secreted by the vagina that varies in consistency.

Vaginal atrophy Thinning of the vaginal walls, which can cause dryness and irritation.

Vaginal oestrogen A form of oestrogen (female hormone) that is administered in the form of a pessary or cream into the vagina.

Virus Simple, small microorganisms that replicate inside cells and can cause disease.

Vulva The external female genitals.

Vulvodynia Pain and discomfort in and around the vulval, vaginal and groin area. Can be generalised or provoked.

Withdrawal method A method to avoid pregnancy when the penis is removed from the vagina before orgasm/ejaculation to prevent sperm entering the vagina.

Womb The non-medical word used to describe the uterus.

X-ray A diagnostic tool that involves passing electromagnetic radiation of short wavelength and high energy through the body to view bones, organs and internal tissues.

RESOURCES

FAIR HEALTHCARE ACCESS FOR ALL
Women's health & disability

Sisters of Frida organization, a collective of disabled women: www.sisofrida.org

Trans patient training for doctors

GPs can access an excellent module on the Royal College of GP's LGBT Health Hub: www.elearning.rcgp.org.uk

The Gender GP online clinic also contains a wealth of useful information for physicians and patients: www.gendergp.com

INFORMATION AND HELP DURING YOUR FERTILITY YEARS
Pregnancy & childbirth

General advice and guidance can be found on these websites:

Tommy's, a pregnancy charity: www.tommys.org

Emma's Diary: www.emmasdiary.co.uk

National Childbirth Trust: www.nct.org.uk/pregnancy

NHS pregnancy advice: www.nhs.uk/pregnancy

Second & third pregnancy trimesters

The following books offer good advice:

The Modern Midwife's Guide to Pregnancy, Birth and Beyond by Marie Louise

Hypnobirthing: Practical Ways to Make Your Birth Better by Siobhan Miller

What to Expect When You're Expecting by Heidi Murkoff

Pregnancy for Men: The Whole Nine Months by Mark Woods

The Expectant Dad's Survival Guide by Rob Kemp

Having a baby if you're LGBT+

NHS advice: www.nhs.uk/pregnancy/having-a-baby-if-you-are-lgbt-plus/

Help with quitting smoking

NHS advice and app: www.nhs.uk/better-health/quit-smoking/

RESOURCES

Health & fitness resources

NHS BMI calculator: www.nhs.uk/live-well/healthy-weight/bmi-calculator

NHS healthy eating guidance: www.nhs.uk/live-well/eat-well/

NHS Couch to 5K: www.nhs.uk/live-well/exercise/running-and-aerobic-exercises/get-running-with-couch-to-5k

My Fitness Pal: www.myfitnesspal.com

Lose It! weight loss plan: www.loseit.com

Eating disorders

BEAT, a charity offering great practical support: www.beateatingdisorders.org.uk

National Centre for Eating Disorders: www.eating-disorders.org.uk

Unplanned pregnancies & ending a pregnancy

Brook, offering confidential advice for young people: www.brook.org.uk

British Pregnancy Advisory Service: www.bpas.org.uk

Pregnancy Crisis Helpline: www.pregnancycrisishelpline.org.uk; Helpline: 0800 368 9296

National Unplanned Pregnancy Advice Service: www.nupas.co.uk

Marie Stopes Clinics for abortion care services: www.msichoices.org.uk

Planned Parenthood, a US-based organization for advice and guidance: www.plannedparenthood.org

Miscarriage support

Tommy's, a pregnancy charity offering support for baby loss: www.tommys.org

Miscarriage Association for miscarriage support: www.miscarriageassociation.org.uk

Sands, support for stillbirth and neonatal loss: www.sands.org.uk

Lullaby Trust, offering emotional support for bereaved families of Sudden Infant Death Syndrome: www.lullabytrust.org.uk

Life After Baby Loss by Nicola Gaskin

Premature birth

Bliss, offering support for babies born premature or sick: www.bliss.org.uk

Ectopic pregnancy

The Ectopic Pregnancy Trust has some really useful information: www.ectopic.org.uk

Pregnancy in Black & ethnic minority communities

RESOURCES

Maternal Mental Health Alliance: www.maternalmentalhealthalliance.org
Black women's maternity experiences report: www.fivexmore.com

PCOS

British and Irish Hypertension Society: www.bihsoc.org
Verity, a PCOS support charity based on Twitter: @veritypcos
PCOS Awareness Association: www.pcosaa.org
PCOS Vitality: www.pcosvitality.com
DAISy-PCOS for PCOS research: www.daisypcos.com
Cysters: www.cysters.org

Endometriosis
Endometriosis UK has a fabulous website for information: www.endometriosis-uk.org

IVF
ICB guidelines and NICE recommendations on NHS in-vitro fertilization (IVF) availability: www.nhs.uk/conditions/ivf/availability
The British Infertility Counselling Association provides advice and guidance to people of all ages who are considering fertility treatment and preservation: www.bica.net
The Fertility Network UK campaigns for equitable access to NHS-funded fertility treatment: www.fertilitynetworkuk.org
Proud 2b Parents, for LGBTQ+ parents seeking IVF advice: www.proud2bparents.co.uk
Stonewall, advice for LGBTQ+ parents: www.stonewall.org.uk

Mental health during pregnancy
Mind: www.mind.org.uk
Tommy's, a pregnancy charity: www.tommys.org
Pandas, perinatal mental illness support: www.pandasfoundation.org.uk

Gynaecological cancer support
Target Ovarian Cancer offers some great tools and resources: www.targetovariancancer.org.uk
The Eve Appeal, a wonderful gynaecological cancer charity: www.eveappeal.org.uk

Breast health & post-cancer care
Breast Cancer Now: www.breastcancernow.org
Macmillan Cancer Support: www.macmillan.org.uk

RESOURCES

CoppaFeel, a breast cancer charity: www.coppafeel.org.uk (also great on Twitter, TikTok and Instagram)

Cancer Research UK: www.cancerresearchuk.org

STATISTICS RESOURCES

Page 42: 8.9% of the residents of England and Wales did not have English as their main language in 2021 (Office for National Statistics 2021 Census, 29 November 2022. www.ons.gov.uk/peoplepopulationandcommunity/culturalidentity/language/bulletins/languageenglandandwales/census2021)

Page 72: 1 in 7 couples in the UK are affected by infertility (NHS data, accessed 1 March 2023. www.nhs.uk/conditions/infertility)

Page 83: 1 in 6 adoptions in England in 2021 were to same-sex couples ('Children looked after in England including adoption: 2020 to 2021, Department for Education Gov.uk website, 18 November 2021. https://www.gov.uk/government/statistics/children-looked-after-in-england-including-adoption-2020-to-2021)

Page 110: Black women in the UK are 4 times more likely to die in pregnancy and childbirth than white women ('Saving Lives, Improving Mothers' Care: Lessons learned to inform maternity care from the UK and Ireland Confidential Enquiries into Maternal Deaths and Morbidity 2017–19', Mothers and Babies: Reducing Risk through Audits and Confidential Enquiries across the UK, November 2021. https://www.npeu.ox.ac.uk/assets/downloads/mbrrace-uk/reports/maternal-report-2021/MBRRACE-UK_Maternal_Report_2021_-_FINAL_-_WEB_VERSION.pdf)

Page 153: By age 35, 60% of Black women are thought to have uterine fibroids, compared to 6% of white women ('Understanding Racial Disparities for Women with Uterine Fibroids' by Beata Mostafavi, Michigan Medicine, University of Michigan website, 12 August 2020. https://www.michiganmedicine.org/health-lab/understanding-racial-disparities-women-uterine-fibroids#:~:text=Nearly%20a%20quarter%20of%20Black,fibroids%20or%20suffer%20from%20complications)

INDEX

INDEX

INDEX

INDEX

ACKNOWLEDGEMENTS

This book and my medical career so far would not have been possible without the help and support of so many people. It's true that it really does take a village! And in particular I'd like to thank the following people and organizations.

I want to say a huge thank you to my family. My parents, whose duas (prayers) and guidance continue to support me, and my siblings, Irfan, Imran, Saba and Ali, who will always be my best friends. My husband, Khalid, is a pillar of support, a dad to our three boys, and a soundboard for the choices I make. To my children, Haris, Qasim and Adam, who are my world and provide so much fun in my life. To the Pakistani women in my community: when I first arrived in the UK, they provided so much food, love, education and embraced us with open arms. These incredible women continue to teach me the facets of womanhood to this day.

When it comes to medicine and women's health, I am fully aware that I stand on the shoulders of giants, in particular Dr Louise Newson, who gave me the courage to push my understanding on HRT and menopause care and translate that to my South Asian community. Dr Annice Mukherjee made me understand the impact of hormones in women, and to Dr Radikha Vohra, Dr Aziza Sesey, Dr Liz O'Riordan, Dr Philippa Kaye, Dr Zoe Williams, Dr Larissa, Dr Sara Hyat, Dr Punam Krishan, Dr Naomi Potter – whose book with Davina McCall I contributed to – thank you for your support. Thank you also to my colleagues from the US from whom I learn so much: Dr Karen Tang, Dr Mary Claire Haver and Dr Rachel Rubin.

To all the people who have contributed towards getting this book into its current state, thank you. In particular, Dr Ajay Verma who has been immensely helpful in providing me with education and support when proofreading sections of the book, and Dr Kamilah Kamaruddin, who is a voice for trans rights in the medical community and gave her wise insight into the sections on healthcare for trans people.

A huge thank you to my family at Wellbeing of Women, especially Dame Lesley Regan, Janet Lindsay, who brought me on as an ambassador, and my fellow ambassador Rosie Nixon, for her constant support. Thanks also to Manjit Gill MBE from Binti Period, whose campaigning about periods is invaluable and who contributed her knowledge about the myths around menstrual cycles, and to Hibo Wardere and Nimko Ali OBE, whose advice helped me to write about FGM with clarity and authority. I'm eternally grateful for grassroots campaigners who do so much for women's health: Diane Danzebrink, founder of Menopause Support; Elizabeth Carr-Ellis From Pausitivity; and South Asian breast cancer campaigns and campaigners, Sakoon Through Cancer, Iyna Butt, Kreena Dhiman and Bep Dhaliwal. And thank you to the charities: The Eve Appeal, Jo's Cervical Cancer Trust, Breast Cancer Now, Lichen Sclerosus and Vulval Cancer UK Awareness who have been a wealth of information and have always supported my work.

Thanks to Jan Croxson, my agent, who found me in 2019, met me for 30 seconds and said she'd like to sign me. I was gobsmacked that somebody would take a punt on a hijab-wearing, slightly potty-mouthed, Muslim woman with three kids and take me into the world of media along with Borra Garson and Louise Leftwich. To Davina McCall for being so supportive and lifter of women.

To Kate Muir who originally asked me to be involved with *Davina McCall: Sex, Myths and the Menopause*. To Eleanor Mills who helped me to write about women's health and who brought me on as an ambassador for Noon.

A huge thank you to the BBC and ITV teams. Thanks also to my BBC Three Counties Radio team, especially Louise Parry, and Toby Friedner, who tried to teach me the art of presenting on a Sunday morning when I've had little to no breakfast and half a cup of tea, but with whom it's been an absolute blast to learn – there is more to presenting than I was ever aware of.

Thank you Baroness Sayeeda Warsi, Saira Khan, Anita Rani, Pippa Vosper, Lavina Mehta MBE, Meera Bhogal, Tessy Ojo CBE, for always championing my work. My HerSpirit friends: Mel Berry, Holly Woodford and Professor Greg Whyte, who literally motivate me to do exercise and get fitter, stronger, healthier in every way because I consume more chocolate than I should!

A huge thank you to my NHS surgery, in particular my supportive colleagues Dr Heather White, Dr Kirsten Riemer and Dr Lee Mitchell. To all my colleagues at OSD Healthcare who helped me set up a private women's health clinic to my own exacting specifications, even getting Entonox for pain relief in my coil insertion clinics. And to my NHS patients, who through their lived experience, have been more of an education than any medical textbook.

A massive thank you to Stephanie Jackson for believing in the vision of this book and taking on this huge gauntlet of a project. I'm so grateful to Jo Lake and Han, whose wisdom and advice I very much appreciated. I'm also grateful to Pauline Bache, Jaz Bahra, and Liliana Rasmussen for all their help, without Liliana's illustrations, this book would not have the soul that it does have.

My teachers at the Misbourne School, in particular my head teacher David Selman, who refused to make me head-girl so I could concentrate on my A-levels and become the first student from the school to go on to study medicine, thank you. Mrs Carol Taylor who provided me with mentorship and tissues as I cried in her office on a practically daily basis for fear of failure (she always had shortbread biscuits and tea); Ms Lorraine Cummings who helped me do my UCAS application to get into Queen Mary's University of London Barts and the London School of Medicine. And to all the professors, friends, lecturers at Barts who put me on my journey to becoming a doctor.

Finally to nine-year-old me, the little Nighat, who was so lost and had left everything she had known in Pakistan. She was in an alien world, never having the right clothing for the wet and cold weather, not understanding the new food and way of life, but she also gained all these freedoms and was able to not be hindered as a girl. Moving here, I felt a bittersweet loss of my life in Pakistan but I also realized a love of what I found in the UK. There's no other place like my hometown of Chesham. When I came here as that young girl I was constantly battling to try and find my identity, so I want to say thank you to that girl, because she persevered with a smile (still, when I'm nervous I smile, which is why I'm always smiling on TV!) and for gradually loosened the shackles of the patriarchy in a small way, being slightly rebellious and finding company in medicine. Because of that, this book is for all the other people who have a sense of loss of identity and loss of grounding – and who every now and then say to themselves, What am I doing? I hope that you can at least feel like you have a handle on and an understanding of your own body and how to best care for it, as a helping hand along the way.

ABOUT THE AUTHOR

Dr Nighat Arif is a GP specializing in women's health and family planning with over 16 years of experience in the NHS and private practice. She is based in Buckinghamshire, UK and is able to consult fluently with patients in Urdu and Punjabi. Dr Nighat is a medical educator and provides teaching to local trainee GPs as well as at national and international conferences. Dr Nighat was nominated for the National Bevan Prize for Health and Wellbeing to acknowledge her exceptional commitment to advancing wellbeing in her community. Dr Nighat has worked to raise awareness on menopause and women's healthcare in Black and Asian women; she presented her clinical work at the 'Menopause in the Workplace' Parliamentary committee hearing. She has also worked with Team Halo, a United Nations (UN) initiative to bring an end to the pandemic and presented at the G7 Global Vaccine Confidence Summit that led to her being awarded an Honorary Doctorate Degree in Science at London City University for Women's Health, Public Health and Inclusion. She is the honorary recipient of the 2023 SHE Award and received a Points of Light Award 2023 from the UK Prime Minister in recognition of her exceptional service to raising awareness for women's health in the UK.

Dr Nighat is the resident doctor on *BBC Breakfast*, ITV'S *This Morning* and BBC *LookEast*, and she hosts her own Sunday Breakfast show on BBC3 Counties

Radio. Dr Nighat was also a contributor on the Channel 4 documentary *Davina McCall: Sex, Lies and the Menopause* and has made guest appearances on numerous podcasts tackling taboos around women's health. Dr Nighat has regularly written for various publications including *Stylist*, *HELLO*, *Red*, *Good Housekeeping* and *Women in Medicine* and her work around menopause has featured in *British Vogue*. She is also an ambassador of the global charity Wellbeing of Women, Roald Dahl's Marvellous Children's Charity, The Good Grief Trust, HerSpirit, Sikh Forgiveness and Upon Noon. She lives in Buckinghamshire with her husband and three sons.

@DrNighatArif